Bibliotherapy

Bibliotherapy

Edited by
**Sarah McNicol
and
Liz Brewster**

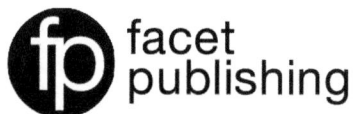

**facet
publishing**

© This compilation: Sarah McNicol and Liz Brewster 2018
The chapters: the contributors 2018

Published by Facet Publishing,
7 Ridgmount Street, London WC1E 7AE
www.facetpublishing.co.uk

Facet Publishing is wholly owned by CILIP: the Library and Information
Association.

British Library Cataloguing in Publication Data
A catalogue record for this book is available from the British Library.

ISBN 978–1–78330–341–0 (paperback)
ISBN 978–1–78330–342–7 (hardback)
ISBN 978–1–78330–343–4 (e-book)

First published 2018

Text printed on FSC accredited material.

Mixed Sources
Product group from well-managed
forests and other controlled sources
www.fsc.org Cert no. SA-COC-1565
© 1996 Forest Stewardship Council
FSC

Typeset from editors' files by Flagholme Publishing Services in 10/14pt Palatino and
Frutiger
Printed and made in Great Britain by CPI Group (UK) Ltd, Croydon, CR0 4YY.

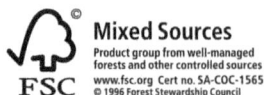

Contents

List of figures and tables

Figures

Tables

Contributors

Elena Azadbakht is an assistant professor and the Heath and Nursing Librarian at the University of Southern Mississippi. Her research interests include user experience (UX), improving library instruction, and, most recently, issues related to research data management. She is an active member of the Medical Library Association.

Fiona Bailey is a bibliotherapist for Midlothian Libraries, in Scotland. Her background includes 15 years of nursing, counselling and liaison work. She is a mixed-media artist and has a Creative Writing MA from Edinburgh Napier University. She writes experimental fiction and non-fiction.

Liz Brewster is a lecturer at Lancaster Medical School, Lancaster University. Her research focuses on experiences of mental health and wellbeing, and particularly on how creative activities such as reading may affect mental health. She has previously worked in academic and public libraries.

David Chamberlain is a Lead Librarian working for the UK National Health Service and has worked as a librarian for 18 years. Previously, he was a Registered Psychiatric Nurse for ten years. He has travelled extensively and has worked in Leicester, New Zealand, Wales and Worcester. He has had seven papers published, with the emphasis on impact and bibliotherapy. David is a Fellow of CILIP.

Cristina Deberti Martins is a graduate in both librarianship and psychology. She is an adult and adolescent psychotherapist specializing in addictions. Cristina has been a bibliotherapist at the Portal Amarillo addiction centre in Montevideo, Uruguay, since 2007. She has published widely and teaches bibliotherapy courses in the public and private sectors. She was previously a lecturer at the Universidad de la República, Montevideo, and is a visiting lecturer at the Universidad Carlos III de Madrid.

Tracy Englert is an associate professor and the Science and Technology Librarian at the University of Southern Mississippi. She is the recipient of several grants focusing on science and technology and is the creator and co-ordinator for the successful Cook Library Science Café series.

Kate Gielgud is Health Information Co-ordinator for TriBorough Libraries and Archives (London Borough of Hammersmith and Fulham; Royal Borough of Kensington and Chelsea; and Westminster City Council) in the UK. She has held this post since 2011. Kate trained at RADA (the Royal Academy of Dramatic Arts) in the 1970s and has worked as a coach on films and directed plays professionally, and was a member of the National Theatre Company in the UK and the Peter Hall Company. She completed a Diploma in the Application of Psychodynamic Theory to the Principles of Counselling at the Westminster Pastoral Foundation in 2001 and has worked as a volunteer counsellor. Her present post at Westminster Libraries is funded by Public Health commissioners within the council to address health inequalities and includes: the promotion of Books on Prescription; running shared reading groups based on the Reader model; developing access to online health information as part of the digital inclusion initiative; and rolling out Make Every Contact training to all council departments.

Elizabeth Mackenzie is a professional member and currently vice-president of the Dance Therapy Association of Australia (DTAA). As co-ordinator of the Activities and Wellbeing programme at St Vincent's Prague House in Melbourne, Elizabeth enjoys bringing an arts- and strengths-based emphasis to recreation and wellbeing activities.

Susan McLaine has travelled to the UK to undertake further research and training in the field of bibliotherapy. Since 2009 she has been initiating Australian developments in bibliotherapy, including developing and co-ordinating the State Library of Victoria's Book Well programme. She has undertaken a PhD study, investigating how facilitators from non-clinical backgrounds can effectively deliver bibliotherapy to support the general wellbeing of individuals and communities.

Sarah McNicol is a research associate at the Education and Social Research Institute, Manchester Metropolitan University. She has worked as an information studies researcher since 2000 and she previously worked as a school librarian. At present, much of her research is focused around the use of graphic comics and novels to explore a range of issues, in particular health and wellbeing.

Natalia Tukhareli received her doctorate in Linguistics from the Moscow State University in Russia and her Master's in Library and Information Science from the University of Western Ontario in Canada. Her professional experience includes service in libraries and non-profit organizations, teaching in post-secondary institutions and scholarly research in various fields. Since 2010, she has been actively involved in bibliotherapy. Natalia has developed and implemented a number of bibliotherapy-based reading programmes to promote wellbeing and resilience to diverse groups of people, including African children and women living with HIV/AIDS, marginalized populations in Toronto, and the staff of a community hospital. Natalia is a published author in both Russian and English. Her scholarly manuscript *Healing Through Books: the evolution and diversification of bibliotherapy* was published in 2014. Currently, she holds the position of Librarian at the Health Sciences Library at Scarborough Rouge Hospital in Toronto, Canada.

Rosie May Walworth is an English literature graduate who works at Rethink Mental Illness in London. Between 2016 and 2018 she worked for The Reading Agency as Programme Assistant, then Acting Programme Manager, on the Reading Well Books on Prescription scheme.

Introduction

The basic premise of bibliotherapy is that information, guidance and solace can be found through reading. Bibliotherapy programmes using books to support good mental health are found around the world. In the UK, programmes such as Reading Well and Books on Prescription have been offered in public libraries, healthcare and community settings since the early 2000s, providing access to selected written materials which, it is hoped, will have a positive effect on mental health. Understandings of bibliotherapy have changed over time and between locations. Whilst many bibliotherapy programmes have traditionally focused on self-help resources, schemes working with fiction and poetry are becoming ever more common. This book will encompass all aspects of 'bibliotherapy' in its widest sense, defined as: 'The therapeutic use of books and other materials with individuals or with groups of people' (Howie, 1988).

The first section of the book consists of four chapters concerned with the history and theory of bibliotherapy. Bibliotherapy draws on theories from a range of disciplines, including medicine, literature, education and psychology. Chapters 1 to 4 draw on just some of these to illustrate some of the contemporary debates amongst researchers interested in bibliotherapy and explain how these relate to the work of bibliotherapy practitioners. These chapters are intended to be of interest not only for researchers and theorists, but equally to those managing bibliotherapy programmes. It is only through developing an understanding of theories underpinning various types of bibliotherapy intervention that practitioners can make informed decisions about which models of bibliotherapy may be most effective for a given setting and audience, as well as appropriate ways to select texts, lead discussions, provide support and so forth. Part 1 therefore links theory and practice: drawing on examples from the case studies in this book and elsewhere to illustrate the key concepts discussed.

In Chapter 1, Liz Brewster highlights some of the major developments since the term 'bibliotherapy' was coined in 1916. The chapter traces the evolution of the models of delivery, types of material used and the diverse audiences for bibliotherapy schemes, reflecting the socio-cultural drivers for its use. Looking back over 100 years of bibliotherapy places it into context and demonstrates why it has continued to be a popular and relevant method of meeting mental health and wellbeing needs.

Chapter 2 outlines some of the theories behind bibliotherapy and demonstrates how they relate to practical bibliotherapy initiatives. It is concerned with not only demonstrating the effectiveness of bibliotherapy, but with understanding *how* it works. This can be a complex area, as there is no single standard approach to bibliotherapy. This chapter therefore considers how theories apply to different types of bibliotherapy found in libraries and other settings. This includes schemes focused on the individual as well as collective activities, and schemes concerned with the consumption of literature as well as those more focused on its creation.

Chapter 3 builds on the theories of bibliotherapy explored in Chapter 2, to consider the relationships between illness narratives, narrative medicine and bibliotherapy. The role of stories told by, and about, people with mental and physical health problems has been underexplored in bibliotherapy practice. The chapter focuses on the theoretical underpinnings of illness narratives and narrative medicine, and contrasts them with current models of bibliotherapy. It concludes that the potential use of stories about health and medicine stretch beyond current bibliotherapy practice and suggests some areas where further links with bibliotherapy may be explored.

Chapter 4 explores the ways in which graphic novels and comics can be used as a form of bibliotherapy. While theories of reading suggest that graphic narratives are highly suited to bibliotherapy activities, both attitudinal and practical barriers limit their use at present. This chapter therefore considers how the medium can be particularly effective in supporting important features of bibliotherapy, such as providing reassurance, connection with others, alternative perspectives, and models of identity. It draws on examples of collections and activities from different library settings to demonstrate some of the ways in which graphic texts can be used in bibliotherapy practice as well as discussing the possible challenges of using graphic narratives for bibliotherapy, and how these could be overcome.

Part 2 of the book is more practically focused, presenting a series of case studies illustrating how particular bibliotherapy approaches can be used across different settings and with a variety of user groups. The case studies presented draw on examples from across a range of settings, including public libraries, academic libraries and healthcare settings. Furthermore, collaboration is a key theme; engaging in bibliotherapy offers librarians key opportunities to collaborate with partners such as healthcare providers and arts organizations.

Current UK models of self-help bibliotherapy and bibliotherapy using fiction and poetry have had great influence on models of bibliotherapy internationally. However, practical implementation can, of course, differ between international contexts, depending on differences in models of health and social care and other factors. The case studies in this book reflect the international spread of bibliotherapy initiatives, including examples from the UK, North and South America and Australasia.

A key focus in this book is on methods of offering bibliotherapy for diverse audiences. In the past, the main audiences for bibliotherapy have tended to be well educated and predominantly white and female. By presenting case studies demonstrating how librarians can engage with more diverse audiences, such as homeless populations, psychiatric patients, speakers of other languages and people living with dementia, this book demonstrates how the appeal of bibliotherapy can be widened, thus contributing to libraries' and other organizations' social inclusion and social justice agendas.

In Chapter 5, Natalia Tukhareli, Librarian at Scarborough and Rouge Hospital, Toronto, Canada, provides an overview of bibliotherapy programmes developed and successfully implemented in library and community settings. Natalia's work with communities including those living with HIV/AIDS in Johannesburg, South Africa, and diverse multicultural communities in Toronto, Canada, has led to the development of a programme that uses fiction, non-fiction and poetry to decrease loneliness and promote wellbeing. This programme is currently used in practice with hospital staff and evaluation of the programme demonstrates the value of books and communication around texts in addressing life's challenges and improving individual and social wellbeing.

Long-term bibliotherapy work can offer stability to people with changing circumstances and provides security to explore issues. In Chapter 6, Fiona Bailey, a Healthy Reading Bibliotherapist for Midlothian Libraries in Scotland, reflects on the advantages and ongoing challenges of bibliotherapy work without a 'clear ending'. This includes exploring ways of maintaining a healthy group dynamic over time, such as the selection of session material, developing trust and group cohesion, supporting creativity and addressing issues around stigma attached to groups for wellbeing by reframing the work in a literary context.

Chapter 7 reflects on the learning from a reading group for people with mental health problems who were homeless or at risk of homelessness. Susan McLaine from the State Library, Victoria, Australia, and Elizabeth Mackenzie, Prague House Activities Co-ordinator, who ran the group, build on read-aloud models used in the UK to consider how the benefits of reading may be shared with this vulnerable group. Using pedagogical theory from adult education, the chapter discusses how integrating reading into the routine of a care facility may help to overcome the stigma and marginalization experienced by those at risk of homelessness.

There is little research on bibliotherapy set within a psychiatric ward or hospital and even less on bibliotherapy in an older adult functional in-patient ward. In Chapter 8, therefore, David Chamberlain, a Lead Librarian working for the National Health Service, discusses the challenges and successes experienced in running a reading group for an older adult in-patient psychiatric ward. He describes the practicalities of introducing bibliotherapy in this context, in particular, partnership working, group structure and selecting texts. David also outlines the reported therapeutic benefits from the perspectives of patients and staff.

While the majority of bibliotherapy work tends to be focused on Western European, North American and Australasian contexts, in Chapter 9 Cristina Deberti Martins, Bibliotherapist-Psychologist at the Portal Amarillo Library in Montevideo, Uruguay, reminds us that there is also important work being carried out elsewhere. This chapter gives an overview of bibliotherapy provision in Uruguay, before focusing on her work at the Portal Amarillo Library with socially vulnerable patients, specifically those with drug-use problems. The programme she describes emphasizes the use of poetry to help individuals who have experienced difficult lives to reclaim their own voices.

In Chapter 10, Rosie May Walworth from The Reading Agency reports on the development and evaluation of Reading Well Books on Prescription for Dementia scheme. The scheme is aimed at people with dementia, their relatives and carers, and anyone who is worried about their memory, with books which provide information and advice, support for living well, advice for relatives and carers and personal stories. This chapter outlines the process of choosing and evaluating relevant books for this diverse audience, highlighting the importance of engaging relevant partners to ensure that the needs of a complex population are met.

In contrast, Chapter 11 explores the use of bibliotherapy with another vulnerable group: young people with mental health and wellbeing issues. Rosie May Walworth shares the experience of setting up the Reading Well for

Young People scheme, which provides 13–to–18–year-olds with advice and information about issues like anxiety, stress and OCD, and difficult experiences such as bullying and exams. The development of the scheme demonstrates how essential it is to work with young people to co-design schemes and use creative responses to encourage discussion between young people about mental health issues.

Chapter 12 focuses on two Read Aloud groups in the London Borough of Westminster: one with a high number of speakers of English as an additional language and the other with predominately highly literate native speakers. In this chapter, Kate Gielgud, Health Information Co-ordinator at Westminster Libraries, considers the group membership and motivations for joining, choice of texts and the role of the facilitator, exploring how these can differ between the two groups.

In Chapter 13, Elena Azadbakht, Health and Nursing Librarian and Tracy Englert, Science & Technology Librarian, both from the University of Southern Mississippi in the USA, describe the development of a Student Success Collection (SSC) encompassing a variety of topics related to student success, such as study skills, career and vocational development, personal development and student life. They discuss the background to this initiative; examine practical aspects such as the location of the collection, stock selection and promotion; and outline possible future directions.

This book therefore demonstrates the potential of bibliotherapy to support diverse groups of people and work across a range of settings: from inpatients, to university students, to those at risk of homelessness. Our aim is that this volume will contribute to ongoing debates about both the theory of bibliotherapy and its practical application. By focusing on the theoretical basis and history of bibliotherapy, as well as current practice, it helps to identify areas in which bibliotherapy could grow as a field of study and of practice.

Reference

Howie M. (1988) Reading therapy and the social worker. In *Reading Therapy* Clark, J.M. and Bostle, E. (eds), The Library Association.

Part 1

History and theory of bibliotherapy

1

Bibliotherapy: a critical history

Liz Brewster

Introduction

Bibliotherapy schemes have been offered in UK public libraries and healthcare and community settings since the early 2000s, providing access to selected written materials which it is hoped will have a positive effect on mental health. These materials have predominantly been self-help resources focused on diagnosed mental health conditions, but some schemes facilitate access to fiction and poetry with a similar aim of improving mental health and wellbeing. These recent incarnations of bibliotherapy draw on a long, varied and international history. Definitions of bibliotherapy have developed in line with changing attitudes and approaches to mental health treatment, and with the evolving role of hospital and public libraries.

Bibliotherapy has developed over the past 100 years, but the premise remains the same: that information, guidance, and solace can be found in books. Some would take this historical account further, referring to the long association between books and their medicinal qualities, with a phrase carved over the door of several ancient libraries, including those at Alexandria and Thebes, usually translated as 'medicine for the soul' (McDaniel, 1956).

This chapter aims to highlight some of the major developments since the term 'bibliotherapy' was coined in 1916. It traces the development of bibliotherapy, examining how it follows the changing roles of hospital, school and public libraries, and explores how attitudes towards physical and mental health have altered. Outlining a critical history of bibliotherapy shows how it has changed over time in response to wider socio-cultural progress. The chapter sketches the characteristics of five eras of bibliotherapy: the coinage and early use of the term; its emergence in the hospital setting; the solidification of the theory and practice and shift of bibliotherapy outside the hospital; building an evidence base around bibliotherapy; and finally more recent work in public libraries and other community settings. Examining key figures in the history of bibliotherapy also demonstrates how the practice has moved from the hospital and the psychiatric unit to the public library and the community setting. Looking back over 100 years of bibliotherapy places it in context and demonstrates why it has continued to be a popular and relevant method of meeting mental health and wellbeing needs.

Early uses of bibliotherapy

The preliminary underpinnings of the concept of bibliotherapy began with the reform of asylums for the mentally ill in the 19th century. Asylum care was residential and long-term, and often involved physical restraint and cruel treatment. Psychiatry at this time was a fledgling discipline, and mental health problems were seen as moral defects rather than as being medically treatable (Porter, 2002). Attitudes to mental health started to change, with the medical profession stepping in to reframe lunatics as patients and asylums as a place for safe restraint rather than incarceration (Shorter, 1997). Before the term bibliotherapy was coined, advocates of the humane treatment of mentally ill patients in asylums recommended reading as part of revised treatment regimens (Weimerskirch, 1965). These advocates, including Samuel Tuke at the Retreat in York, Philippe Pinel at the Bicêtre Hospital in Paris and Americans Benjamin Rush and John Minson Galt, could not be described as pioneers of bibliotherapy as it would be recognized today. But these considerations of reading as beneficial for the wellbeing of the insane started to shape perceptions and guide the direction of future interventions.

The term 'bibliotherapy' itself was coined in Samuel McCord Crothers' article 'A Literary Clinic' in the journal *Atlantic Monthly* in 1916 (Crothers, 1916). Crothers, an American Unitarian minister and essayist, gave a tongue-in-cheek account of a friend who was using literature to treat patients' existential ills. He took the image of books as having medicinal properties to extend the metaphor for 'a proper prescription' for literary fiction, with his friend running a clinic-bookshop which recommended titles to patients based on their diagnosis. The aim was to cure the reader of all their ills using books rather than pills and ointments. Books were seen as a more acceptable vehicle for treatment, an 'excipient, to make it suitable for administration and pleasant to the patient' (Crothers, 1916, 293). Christopher Morley's novella *The Haunted Bookshop* (1919) also includes one of the first uses of the term bibliotherapy. Morley built on Crothers' metaphor, using imagery of bookshops haunted by the ghosts of 'great literature'. Again in his work, booksellers were providing bibliotherapy to readers in need of literary medicine: 'malnutrition of the reading faculty is a serious thing. Let us prescribe for you' (Morley, 1919, 2).

From these allusions in early-20th-century popular culture, it is clear that books were seen as something with the power to shape minds and heal hearts. However, in the intervening 100 years between early usage and the present day, there have been many interpretations of what constitutes bibliotherapy, who should deliver it and how it should be delivered. Bibliotherapy has a diverse history which encompasses its role in education and information provision, therapy, self-development, reading for pleasure and catharsis. It will be explored here in its widest sense, taking in definitions as they acquired meaning and changed.

Hospital librarianship and bibliotherapy in the World Wars

Along with physical injuries, 'war neurosis' affected a significant number of men who returned from World War I between 1914 and 1918 (Shephard, 2002). Though it is difficult to estimate the exact number of cases of mental stress and distress, the commonality of 'shell shock' and the rapid rise in the number of men with psychological trauma at this time led to new understandings of what caused mental health issues and new approaches to treating problems (Bourke, 2000; Shephard, 2002). Physiological explanations of mental health issues, the idea that a person could break down under stress, were more broadly accepted and psychotherapy expanded as an appropriate treatment.

Occupational therapy, or interventions to support patients with activities with a view to getting them back to everyday life, was still in early development at this time. Instead, hospitals relied on libraries and librarians to keep patients engaged with the world outside the hospital. This often involved providing books which gave patients guidance on developing new skills or interests, which was defined by Dorothy Hoskins Smith, a hospital librarian, as 'remotivation' (Alston, 1962). Most of the focus at this time in the UK and USA appears to have been on enthusiastic hospital librarians who wanted to improve mental health outcomes for their patients. Sadie Peterson Delaney, librarian at the Veterans' Administration hospital in Alabama, championed the importance of reading and of including patients in the administration of library tasks, citing cases of disturbed shell-shocked patients recovering enough to work in the hospital library (Peterson Delaney, 1938). Bibliotherapy at this time was conducted as one-to-one recommendations for patients, or as a group discussion, though its focus was not on providing information about recovery. Edward Alston quotes the suggestion from the era that:

> . . . a mere series of 12 group conversations about such objective topics as fishing, rail-roads, cotton, rock gardens, or cooking, conducted in an atmosphere of friendliness and approval, can give mental patients a strong thrust toward recovery. (Alston, 1962 p.172)

Attempts to categorize bibliotherapy beyond the idea of 'selected reading' did not achieve consensus at this time; questions were asked as to whether bibliotherapy should be provided by clinical or non-clinical staff (such as librarians), or focused on information provision, education and personal development or distraction therapy. The growth of psychotherapy meant that what was considered to be bibliotherapy also developed and books were a potentially useful tool. A major influence in the development of bibliotherapy in the 1930s was psychologist and librarianship scholar Dr Alice Bryan. In 1939, she asked the question: 'can there be a science of bibliotherapy?', theorizing that there were six objectives to selecting reading to work with a patient with psychological difficulties. She connected reading with ideas of identification, motivation, personal values and experience, moving away from ideas of distraction or remotivation and towards a concept of self-understanding (Bryan, 1939). Bryan also called for a more scientific approach to research on bibliotherapy and championed the role of the librarian-as-psychologist in providing this guidance (Dufour, 2014).

Bibliotherapy's alignment with psychology continued, with Caroline Shrodes publishing the first doctoral thesis on the subject (Shrodes, 1949). Shrodes was influenced by the psychoanalytical work of Sigmund Freud, as well as Louise Rosenblatt's (1938) work on Reader Response Theory. Shrodes identified five psychological reactions to reading literature – identification, transference, catharsis, insight and the relation of self to others – and tried to put a framework in place for working with literature to deliver therapeutic outcomes. However, though widely cited, Shrodes' approach was difficult to put into practice for librarians and even psychotherapists (Cohen, 1994; Dufour, 2014). Throughout the 1940s and 1950s, bibliotherapy remained popular and was seen as an effective intervention, but with these notable exceptions there was little theoretical interest in *how* and *why* it worked.

Developing bibliotherapy: resurgence and diversification

Interest in bibliotherapy peaked in the 1960s and 1970s, with an increasing number of books and academic articles published on the subject. As mental health treatment continued to develop, with psychopharmacology as a growing field, the need for institutionalization for mental health issues declined (Shorter, 1997). For scholars and practitioners at the time, this suggested an increasing role for bibliotherapy. Two key publications in the 1960s and 1970s highlighted the ongoing relevance in bibliotherapy and attempts to theorize its effects. First, the 1962 special issue of the journal *Library Trends* brought together scholars and practitioners to explore – amongst other things – the relationship of bibliotherapy to psychotherapy, the role of the librarian and the scale and scope of practice (Alston, 1962; Hannigan, 1962; Jackson, 1962). Edited by Ruth M. Tews, who also wrote the introduction, the special issue highlighted some ongoing issues with bibliotherapy in practice, including the need to clarify its aims, and again called for in-depth research on the topic (Tews, 1962).

Second, Rhea J. Rubin's work in the late 1970s brought together a narrative history of the development of bibliotherapy to this point, collating sources from the literature in support of her argument that bibliotherapy was effective at improving mental health and wellbeing (Rubin, 1978a; 1978b). Rubin (1978b, 4–5) defined three different types of bibliotherapy, which represented the key elements of practice at this time. Her classification also highlights changing attitudes to mental health and wellbeing, showing a fledgling recognition of the continuum or spectrum of mental health. For Rubin, institutional bibliotherapy was located only in the mental institution (as asylums were now commonly known). This form of bibliotherapy had similarities to earlier constructions of bibliotherapy as distraction and/or remotivation; it worked with individuals and aimed to provide information, recreation and re-socialization. What Rubin referred to as clinical bibliotherapy used imaginative literature in groups, either in the mental institution or in the community, and aimed to encourage insight and behavioural change. Finally, developmental bibliotherapy used imaginative literature to maintain good mental health with people who did not have any diagnosis of mental health problems.

In the early history of bibliotherapy (pre-1940s), books used were often fiction or non-fiction unconnected to mental health. As the field developed, librarians were more likely to try to classify books to try to recommend them for particular themes or diagnoses. For example, Rubin (1978b) recommended books for people who need help with decision-making, courage and despair.

Another notable development was that these book lists also included materials for children and young people as well as adults (Brown, 1975; Rubin, 1978b). Using books to explain difficult concepts such as death to children, as well as working in schools, colleges and other settings, including correctional facilities, remained popular on the North American continent.

Much research evidence at this time was of low quality and often rested on the perceived improvements to mental health and wellbeing as understood by the psychotherapist. The focus on anecdote and case report as research led to attempts to establish structures around bibliotherapy, with calls for certification and training (Hynes, 1975; Rubin, 1978b). While bibliotherapy was almost universally regarded as a positive thing, little was understood about how and why it worked and how best to administer it. Rubin's conclusion at the time was:

> . . . current research, it is obvious, is conflicting and confusing. The field is badly in need of further studies which will investigate the effects of bibliotherapy on attitudes towards people and concepts, on attitudes toward behaviour, and on behaviour itself.'
>
> (Rubin, 1978b, 55)

Other library practitioners and academics, such as Beatty (1962) and Sclabassi (1973), also agreed that one of the main issues with bibliotherapy was that it was underdeveloped as a field of research.

Building an evidence base around bibliotherapy

A common theme throughout the history of bibliotherapy in practice is the call for more research, and research of better quality, to demonstrate the impact and effect of bibliotherapy. In particular, the position of bibliotherapy at the edge of medical practice – was it a psychological therapy, a treatment, or a reading intervention? – led to a desire to assess bibliotherapy as a medical intervention, using the rigorous testing methods developed for assessing the effectiveness of medication. Measuring improvements in symptoms became a goal for researchers, and testing the effectiveness of medical and psychological interventions using the randomized controlled trial (RCT) approach become more common. When applied to bibliotherapy, the RCT generally tried to demonstrate that reading a particular book led to statistically significant clinical improvements in symptoms of diagnosed mental health problems.

Often, the books in question were written versions of psychotherapeutic courses of treatment which were established as effective when delivered by a psychotherapist. RCTs then tried to ascertain whether it was necessary to have therapist involvement in the process, with a control group having treatment as usual (TAU) for a mental health issue (e.g. therapist contact/waiting list/medication); a treatment group being given written informational materials and exercises (bibliotherapy only); and a third arm of the trial being given written materials and the support of a psychotherapist (bibliotherapy + TAU). Often this approach to bibliotherapy is known as self-help.

As the evidence base around using written materials within therapeutic approaches grew, several important themes emerged. First, that self-help bibliotherapy approaches were often more effective when facilitated by a therapist or other professional or para-professional (Farrand et al., 2008; Gellatly et al., 2007). One explanation for this increased effectiveness might be that the repeated contact and encouragement might increase the motivation of the person undertaking the treatment to continue with it. There are concerns that this may have led to overestimations of the effectiveness of bibliotherapy without facilitation (Febbraro, 2005). Despite this evidence, many current UK bibliotherapy schemes do not operate a facilitated model.

A second finding was that bibliotherapeutic approaches were more effective when undertaken voluntarily, with the patient choosing bibliotherapy over another treatment, rather than being assigned to bibliotherapy within an RCT (Bergsma, 2008). Bibliotherapy was also more effective when people complied with the recommended treatment (Kupshik and Fisher, 1999). For example, one study examining the use of bibliotherapy with parents aiming to improve child behaviour found that mothers read on average nine out of the ten chapters in the recommended book, with fathers reading on average one chapter. The findings of the study showed that mothers also reported a more significant improvement in their child's behaviour, potentially indicating that their reading had enabled them to implement recommended techniques to improve behaviour (Hahlweg et al., 2008).

However, many studies did not capture *how* and *when* patients used the self-help materials prescribed as treatment within their outcome measures (Bower, Richards and Lovell, 2001; Bowman, Scogin and Lyrene, 1995). This meant that while people got better, it was hard to say that this was because they had read the book and taken the self-help techniques on board. Not asking questions about reading also removed the subjective experience of what it was like to read the books from the narrative and evidence around bibliotherapy. In most studies, the only information provided about the text is the number of pages in the book and a quantified reading age, meaning that it is difficult to assess the importance of linguistic style, therapeutic approach and balance of instruction and reflection that facilitates effective treatment.

Third, using bibliotherapy removed some barriers to traditional mental health treatment. Being able to access a book on mental health problems was less stigmatizing than visiting a medical professional (Cuijpers, 1997). Access to written materials was also more freely available than access to psychotherapeutic treatments, which were often only available at certain locations (often referred to as a geographical barrier to healthcare), at significant cost or after a long waiting period (Mataix-Cols and Marks, 2006; Reeves and Stace, 2005; Richards, 2004). Taking a self-help approach to accessing mental health therapies was also seen to be empowering and provided choice to people who may not have wanted a pharmacological treatment (Clarke et al., 2006; Mains and Scogin, 2003).

Fourth, it became apparent that providing evidence of the long-term effectiveness of bibliotherapy was not a simple process. Evidence-based medicine relies on having a control group for treatment, but its principles also emphasize that if a treatment is thought to be beneficial then it is unethical to withhold that treatment from the control group. Often this leads to use of a 'delayed treatment' group as a control group (for example in Ackerson et al., 1998). Delaying treatment rather than withholding it meant that the longer-term effects of bibliotherapy in comparison with no treatment or TAU are difficult to observe or assess. One trial, examining the impact of bibliotherapy for anxiety for those on waiting lists for therapy, did review relapse and further treatment after three years and found that bibliotherapy was still having a positive effect on the experience of symptoms of mental health problems, but this trial was relatively small and many patients were lost to follow-up (White, 1995; 1998). Addressing questions of long-term effectiveness, relapse and recovery is problematic for all complex interventions for mental health problems, and may demonstrate why the RCT model is not the most appropriate way to address these queries.

Finally, the construction of a broader evidence base also identified an important problem with bibliotherapy: that while using books as a supportive therapy was sound in principle, this did not mean that every book could be regarded as effective. This principle was identified after a review of computer-based therapeutic resources by the UK's National Institute of Health and Care Excellence (NICE). This review concluded that results from RCTs of different computer-based therapeutic resources could only be generalized if all therapeutic resources were regarded as the same and of equal value

(Richardson, Richards and Barkham, 2008). As this is not the case, and the computer-based therapeutic resources all had different patterns of delivery, therapeutic underpinnings and exercises within them, the evidence from one trial only supported the effectiveness of one resource, not all resources. It is clear that the same principle applies to books and written resources trialled, which also vary greatly. A further complication is that the majority of written resources tested in RCTs in the 1990s and 2000s tended not to be commercially published and widely available. This means that access to written materials that have been demonstrated to be effective in trials is actually limited – researchers tend to trial materials that they have written themselves, which are not always subsequently made available. There have been some published studies testing commercially-available products including classic texts on depression, though this has not been a commonplace occurrence (Ackerson et al., 1998).

However, building this evidence base did highlight how versatile bibliotherapy was and how it could be used effectively. For example, bibliotherapy could be used as a precursor to treatment, or while waiting for other treatment. It could also be used as an adjunct to therapy or medication or as a follow-on after other treatment (Kenwright, 2010). Using bibliotherapy removed barriers to treatment, as books were a low-cost, portable solution, and the number of credible studies which demonstrated good outcomes continued to grow (Chamberlain, Heaps and Robert, 2008; Fanner and Urquhart, 2008; Williams and Martinez, 2008). For example, meta-analyses which draw together RCTs to pool effect size and draw more significant conclusions showed that there were statistically significant positive effects on the participants in RCTs of bibliotherapy (Bower, Richards and Lovell, 2001).

Books on Prescription and UK public libraries

The growing evidence around self-help bibliotherapy encouraged a new model, which was first taken forward into UK public libraries in the early 2000s. The first Books on Prescription schemes began in Wales, with a pilot scheme in public libraries in Cardiff in 2003 and UK-wide roll-out in 2005. It quickly became the most widely used model of bibliotherapy in the UK, with over 100 public library authorities having a scheme. In 2013, the scheme was revised and relaunched by a charity, The Reading Agency, as Reading Well Books on Prescription and is currently offered by 97% of English public libraries. It has been part of the Society of Chief Librarians' Public Library Universal Health Offer since 2013.

Books on Prescription was designed to provide a list of self-help titles recommended by mental health professionals in a format that could be easily accessed through public library services. General practitioners (GPs) and other health professionals could prescribe the books to patients they felt might benefit, via a paper prescription system, with the books then available to borrow from the local public library. The list mainly included books with cognitive behavioural therapy techniques on a number of specific conditions, including depression, anxiety and stress. Run in partnership between public library authorities and local health services, the aim was to recommend a specific book to a patient whom health professionals felt would benefit from trialling the techniques and approach laid out in the written resource. Library users could also self-prescribe these titles, choosing to borrow them from the public library without a prescription.

The introduction of Books on Prescription was informed, in part, by the NICE recommended guidelines for treatment for depression, anxiety and bulimia nervosa (National Institute for Health and Care Excellence, 2004a; 2004b; 2004c; 2009). NICE's recommendation of written resources for treatment in these conditions, combined with the low set-up costs of delivering these resources via the public library, was seen as a strong incentive for trialling this approach. Access to psychological therapies in the UK at this time was limited and psychiatrist Dr Neil Frude, who initially suggested partnering public libraries with medical professionals, was passionate in his vision that Books on Prescription would help more people to get the psychological support they needed (Frude, 2004; 2005; 2008). Psychological interventions are more popular with patients than medication, so taking this approach demonstrates treatment acceptability. Books are durable, inexpensive and can be accessed by multiple library users, so the Books on Prescription model was seen as a cost-effective option.

In many ways, Books on Prescription harked back to the bibliotherapy of the 1970s, aiming to provide access to a list of recommended titles for different issues and conditions in life. Frude initially consulted clinical psychiatrists and psychologists to form the list of recommended books, which differed in approach from previous lists of recommended resources that tended to be compiled by librarians or library academics (Clifford, Norcross and Sommer, 1999; Johnson, 1998; Rubin, 1978b). Books on Prescription was designed to meet treatment access issues for people with low-level mental health problems – what Reading Well Books on Prescription now refers to as common mental health conditions – providing an opportunity to access some support while on waiting lists for further treatment or following a referral from secondary care. Because the books all aim to provide support for one defined condition, there are difficulties in recommending them for people with co-morbidities (e.g. with depression and anxiety).

Initial analysis of borrowing figures showed that there was a high demand for these titles, and responses to the annual national evaluation continues to suggest high levels of satisfaction with the scheme (Hicks, 2006; Porter et al., 2006; The Reading Agency, Society of Chief Librarians and BOP Consulting, 2016). However, while this ongoing evaluation demonstrated that those who completed the survey felt that their understanding of their mental health problem and their confidence around managing the condition had improved, it has proved difficult to demonstrate an overall impact in terms of symptom reduction or decreased burden on mental health services.

Other research has contributed to understanding perspectives on Books on Prescription, with several librarianship and psychology dissertations and doctoral theses taking a qualitative approach to analysis of librarian, health professional and library-user views of the schemes and recommended titles (Brewster, 2008; 2011; Furness and Casselden, 2012; Grundy, 2005). Public librarians consulted on their involvement in the early incarnation of Books on Prescription were broadly positive about the approach but expressed some concerns about its delivery in practice (Brewster, 2007). Many of the books on initial Books on Prescription schemes were seen as out-of-date or less appropriate to their community needs. Often books had a very high reading age, making them less accessible to readers with lower literacy levels, and a lack of suitable resources in community languages was noted (Brewster, 2007). Grundy's (2005) research found that readers disliked the American tone of some books, with references to dollars and vacations rather than pounds and holidays, meaning they found it difficult to identify with the books. There was a feeling from public librarians at this time that there was a need for greater involvement of medical professionals at the point of prescription to ensure success. As the scheme has developed, the collections have been refreshed and there has been greater consultation with readers as well as library and clinical professionals to ensure the recommended resources meet identified needs.

However, engagement with medical professionals has still proven to be elusive. In a recent survey, there was limited response from those prescribing the books to patients (The Reading Agency, Society of Chief Librarians and BOP Consulting, 2016). The high number of self-prescriptions in comparison with the number of prescriptions from GPs – along with comments from librarians noted in the evaluation survey – shows the difficulties in engaging GPs in new initiatives outside the health sector.

Under its recent guise, the Reading Well Books on Prescription scheme has expanded from common mental health conditions for adults. There is also a recommended collection of fiction and self-help titles for people with dementia, their families and carers which launched in 2015 and is discussed in Chapter 10. For young people aged 13–18 there is also a collection of self-help titles, with some recommended fiction known as Shelf Help, which similarly covers topics including confidence and self-esteem, anxiety and bullying. This is discussed in Chapter 11. In July 2017, The Reading Agency also launched a collection of Books on Prescription titles for people with long-term conditions including diabetes, heart disease and arthritis. This collection was co-produced with people with experience of living with long-term conditions and also includes titles covering specific symptoms such as pain and fatigue. The inclusion of titles chosen by readers with experience of the conditions under discussion represents another evolution within bibliotherapy, with the expertise of patients and readers recognized as a legitimate source of knowledge.

Reading fiction as therapy

Evidence and practice

As the evidence base around self-help bibliotherapy continued to grow, showing that books could be a good way of providing information and advice on dealing with mental health issues, there was also interest in improving the evidence base around bibliotherapy using fiction and poetry. One issue here is that taking an evidence-based medicine approach to analysing the effect of fiction and poetry is difficult and, some have argued, inappropriate.

Dysart-Gale (2008), for example, critiqued the application of the approach as biased towards biomedical outcomes such as symptom reduction, which meant that the use of RCTs ignores the reader's experience of the literature. While Dysart-Gale was not arguing for a return to low-quality anecdotal research, she questioned the focus on standardized psychological tests to demonstrate the outcome of bibliotherapy with little focus on the books themselves. In common with other creative therapies – writing, art, drama, photography – bibliotherapy based on expression of emotion and self-under-standing struggled to find a language in which health professionals could understand its potential impact. As Forrest (1998) concluded, it was difficult to say that this form of bibliotherapy was evidence-based at all. However, it could be argued that while the biomedical paradigm focuses on an evidence base subscribing to these standards, few schemes and interventions, if any, delivered in libraries are tested in RCTs and knowledge claims do not rely on this model. While there have been calls for evidence-based librarianship (Booth, 2003), in practice the quality of evidence is usually limited by a need to understand the impact of a scheme in a quick and cost-effective manner. Instead, librarianship focuses on a more realist paradigm of knowledge – what works for whom and in what circumstances (Pawson, 2006).

Reading fiction as therapy in UK public libraries

The early 2000s was a growth time for different types of bibliotherapy in the UK. Using reading as a creative therapy also became popular in public libraries and health services. Although not as widespread as the Books on Prescription scheme, approaches to group reading and shared reading for wellbeing have become well established and the evidence base around the models currently in use continues to grow. In the north of England, Kirklees Public Library Service employed three bibliotherapists in 2000, who had responsibility for promoting reading for wellbeing: running groups and events and working with individuals to engage them with reading and the public library service. Initially known as the Reading and You Scheme (RAYS), the scheme aimed to encourage people to use books and reading for wellbeing and to relax. Now known as Well into Words, the scheme works in public libraries, day services and in-patient wards for people with mental health issues or dementia. The model encompasses many different elements (Morral, 2016), including:

- shared reading groups, in which the group read a text together in the group setting and discuss
- groups similar to traditional reading groups, in which readers meet to discuss a previously-read book
- creative writing groups, in which people read and discuss their own poetry and writing as well as that of others
- individual bibliotherapy, where a bibliotherapist provides support one-to-one, sometimes as a precursor to joining a reading group
- bibliotexting, which shares poetry or quotations via text message to a group mailing list.

The poetry and fiction used in Kirklees is very diverse and initially there was not a list of recommended titles for bibliotherapeutic work. Instead, the bibliotherapists worked with the needs of individuals and groups to connect readers with books. In 2009, with the aim of spreading their expertise further, they published a *Bibliotherapy Toolkit* which contained advice on how to run a creative bibliotherapy group and a preliminary list of fiction and poetry that might engage readers (Duffy et al., 2009).

The early 2000s were a fertile time for new models of bibliotherapy using fiction and poetry in the UK. The Reader, an organisation which promotes the enjoyment of reading, was founded by Jane Davis, an English teacher working in the Department of Continuing Education at the University of Liverpool. Davis designed a shared reading intervention initially called Get Into Reading and now known as Shared Reading (Longden et al., 2015). Her intention was to encourage people to engage with and enjoy 'classic' literature that they might not otherwise have read, with a view that the universal themes within this type of literature could speak to all. The vision is partly educational and partly about improving wellbeing – giving people the skills and confidence to read, discuss and relate literature to their lives. The model rested on shared reading groups, initially run in public libraries, day centres and in-patient wards, including secure mental health settings, in Merseyside in the UK.

The Reader predominantly uses literary work that it refers to as 'great literature', including George Eliot, Doris Lessing, Jane Austin, William Shakespeare and Charles Dickens (Dowrick et al., 2012). With its basis in English and education, The Reader places value judgements on fiction and poetry with which not all may agree. Nevertheless, its approach has been popular and successful. The Reader became an independent charity in 2008, having previously been commissioned to work with health services and in public libraries. The Reader's Shared Reading model has spread nationally and internationally, with a focus on providing training and volunteer-led projects as well as delivering Shared Reading in diverse settings such as the Northern Irish prison system.

Alongside its community work, The Reader also collaborates with the Centre for Research into Reading, Literature and Society at the University of Liverpool, which works to investigate the relationship between arts, health and mental health, the theoretical bases for bibliotherapy, and evaluates the impact of literature-based interventions. This academic work has helped to diversify and improve the evidence base for using fiction and poetry as therapy, taking research techniques from health and medicine, the social sciences and the humanities to make links between reading and wellbeing (Billington et al., 2010; Dowrick et al., 2012; Longden et al., 2015; O'Sullivan et al., 2015).

Interest in using fiction and poetry as a form of bibliotherapy is also shown in The Reading Agency's annual list of *Mood Boosting Books*. Chosen by readers and reading groups, the aim is to provide a selection of titles that are uplifting. Again, it is difficult to evaluate the impact of this scheme on people with mental health conditions, but attempts to synthesize the evidence base around using fiction and poetry conclude that it can contribute to increased cultural and social capital. This recent report, commissioned by The Reading Agency (The Reading Agency and BOP Consulting, 2015), reviewed the impact of reading for pleasure and empowerment. It concluded that as much of the research had been conducted recently, in the last five years, there needs to be a stronger evidence base around this emergent field. Although this chapter has shown the long history of bibliotherapy in practice, in many ways the history of research around bibliotherapy is just beginning. In particular, opportunities for longitudinal work, following up people who have used bibliotherapy schemes to look at the longer-term impact on their wellbeing and reading, have only just started to emerge.

Conclusion

Overall, this chapter has shown that understandings of bibliotherapy have changed over time and in different locations. The diversity of approach has been reflected in questions around who should lead bibliotherapy initiatives and what their involvement should be; who should choose the books included; and what focus they should have. From the hospital library providing distraction therapy to wounded military personnel, bibliotherapy schemes have evolved and now engage with public libraries' role within the wider community. The history of bibliotherapy also reflects the changing understanding of mental health and wellbeing, as well as changes in treatment and, more broadly, approaches to medicine. As mental health conditions have become more de-stigmatized and there has been a shift away from institutionalized treatment, bibliotherapy has also evolved.

At the same time, the quality of evidence required to establish the effectiveness of bibliotherapy has also changed, with the need to establish defined and tangible outcomes from investment in these schemes. The high number of people in the UK self-referring to schemes like Reading Well Books on Prescription and working with The Reader show that bibliotherapy still has a role to play in helping people to secure their mental health and wellbeing through reading. As public library services adapt, change and consider new service models, this chapter has shown that they should still consider placing bibliotherapy at the heart of what they do.

As will be seen in Part 2 of this book, current UK models of self-help bibliotherapy and bibliotherapy using fiction and poetry have had great influence on current models of bibliotherapy internationally. Books on Prescription is available in many public libraries in the USA, and The Reader's Shared Reading model has been adopted in Australia, Belgium, the Netherlands, Germany and Denmark. The broadly Western European, North American and Australasian focus to bibliotherapy work may not reflect attitudes to mental health throughout the wider world. Spreading bibliotherapy more widely as the evidence base around it continues to grow may be the next step in bibliotherapy's history.

References

Ackerson, J., Scogin, F., McKendree-Smith, N. and Lyman, R. D. (1998) Cognitive Bibliotherapy for Mild and Moderate Adolescent Depressive Symptomatology, *Journal of Consulting and Clinical Psychology*, **66** (4), 685–90.

Alston, E. F. (1962) Bibliotherapy and Psychotherapy, *Library Trends*, **11** (2), 159–76.

Beatty, W. K. (1962) A Historical Review of Bibliotherapy, *Library Trends*, **11** (2), 106–17.

Bergsma, A. (2008) Do Self-help Books Help?, *Journal of Happiness Studies*, **9** (3), 341–360.

Billington, J., Dowrick, C., Robinson, J., Hamer, A. and Williams, C. (2010) An Investigation into the Therapeutic Benefits in Relation to Depression and Wellbeing, University of Liverpool and Liverpool Primary Care Trust, www.thereader.org.uk/investigation-therapeutic-benefits-reading-relation-depression-well.

Booth, A. (2003) Bridging the Research-Practice Gap? The role of evidence based librarianship, *New Review of Information and Library Research*, **9** (1), 3–23.

Bourke, J. (2000) Effeminacy, Ethnicity and the End of Trauma: the sufferings of 'shell-shocked' men in Great Britain and Ireland 1914–39, *Journal of Contemporary History*, **35** (1), 57–69.

Bower, P., Richards, D. and Lovell, K. (2001) The Clinical and Cost-effectiveness of Self-help Treatments for Anxiety and Depressive Disorders in Primary Care: a systematic review, *British Journal of General Practice*, **51** (471), 838–45.

Bowman, D., Scogin, F. R. and Lyrene, B. (1995) The Efficacy of Self-examination Therapy and Cognitive Bibliotherapy in the Treatment of Mild to Moderate Depression, *Psychotherapy Research*, **5** (2), 131–40.

Brewster, L. (2007) (Brewster, E. A.) *'Medicine for the Soul': bibliotherapy and the public library*, MA thesis, University of Sheffield, http://dagda.shef.ac.uk/dispub/dissertations/2006-07/External/Brewster_ Elizabeth_MALib.pdf.

Brewster, L. (2008) Medicine for the Soul, *Public Library Journal*, **23** (2), 5–7.

Brewster, L. (2011) (Brewster, E. A.) *An Investigation of Experiences of Reading for Mental Health and Wellbeing and their Relation to Models of Bibliotherapy*, PhD thesis, University of Sheffield, http://etheses.whiterose.ac.uk/2006.

Brown, E. F. (1975) *Bibliotherapy and its Widening Application*, Scarecrow Press.

Bryan, A. (1939) Can There be a Science of Bibliotherapy?, *Library Journal*, **64**, 773–6.

Chamberlain, D., Heaps, D. and Robert, I. (2008) Bibliotherapy and Information Prescriptions: a summary of the published evidence-base and recommendations from past and ongoing Books on Prescription projects, *Journal of Psychiatric and Mental Health Nursing*, **15** (1), 24–36.

Clarke, G., Lynch, F., Spofford, M. and De Barr, L. (2006) Trends Influencing Future Delivery of Mental Health Services in Large Healthcare Systems, *Clinical Psychology*, **13** (3), 287–92.

Clifford, J. S., Norcross, J. C. and Sommer, R. (1999) Autobiographies of Mental Health Clients: psychologists' use and recommendations, *Professional Psychology – Research & Practice*, **30** (1), 56–9.

Cohen, L. (1994) The Experience of Therapeutic Reading, *Western Journal of Nursing Research*, **16** (4), 426–37.

Crothers, S. M. (1916) A Literary Clinic, *Atlantic Monthly*, **118**, 291–301.

Cuijpers, P. (1997) Bibliotherapy in Unipolar Depression: a meta-analysis, *Journal of Behaviour Therapy and Expressive Psychiatry*, **28** (2), 139–47.

Dowrick, C., Billington, J., Robinson, J., Hamer, A. and Williams, C. (2012) Get into Reading as an Intervention for Common Mental Health Problems: exploring catalysts for change. *Medical Humanities* **38** (1), 15–20.

Duffy, J., Haslam, J., Holl, L., and Walker, J. (2009) *Bibliotherapy Toolkit*, Kirklees Council, https://www.scribd.com/document/214685513/Bibliotherapy-Toolkit

Dufour, M. S. (2014) *Reading for Health: bibliotherapy and the medicalized humanities in the United States, 1930–1965*, Virginia Polytechnic Institute and State University, https://vtechworks.lib.vt.edu/handle/10919/65149.

Dysart-Gale, D. (2008) Lost in Translation: bibliotherapy and evidence-based medicine, *Journal of Medical Humanities*, **29** (1), 33–43.

Fanner, D. and Urquhart, C. (2008) Bibliotherapy for Mental Health Service Users Part 1: a systematic review, *Health Information and Libraries Journal*, **25** (4), 237–52.

Farrand, P., Confue, P., Byng, R. and Shaw, S. (2008) Guided Self-help Supported by Paraprofessional Mental Health Workers: an uncontrolled before-after cohort study, *Health and Social Care in the Community*, **17** (1), 9–17.

Febbraro, G. (2005) An Investigation into the Effectiveness of Bibliotherapy and

Minimal Contact Interventions in the Treatment of Panic Attacks, *Journal of Clinical Psychology*, **61** (6), 763–79.

Forrest, M. E. S. (1998) Recent Developments in Reading Therapy: a recent review of the literature, *Health Libraries Review*, **15** (2), 157–64.

Frude, N. (2004) A Book Prescription Scheme in Primary Care, *Clinical Psychology*, **39**, 11–14.

Frude, N. (2005) Prescription for a Good Read, *Healthcare Counselling and Psychotherapy Journal*, **5** (1), 9–13.

Frude, N. (2008) Book Prescriptions: five years on, *Healthcare Counselling and Psychotherapy Journal*, **9**, 8–10.

Furness, R. and Casselden, B. (2012) An Evaluation of a Books on Prescription Scheme in a UK Public Library Authority, *Health Information and Libraries Journal*, **29** (4), 333–7.

Gellatly, J., Bower, P., Hennessy, S., Richards, D., Gilbody, S. and Lovell, K. (2007) What Makes Self-help Interventions Effective in the Management of Depressive Symptoms? Meta-analysis and meta-regression, *Psychological Medicine*, **37** (9) 1217–28.

Grundy, L. (2005) *Evaluation of the 'Cardiff Book Prescription Scheme': prescription of self-help books for people with mild to moderate mental health problems*, Cardiff University, http://ethos.bl.uk/OrderDetails.do?uin=uk.bl.ethos.494481.

Hahlweg, K., Heinrichs, N., Kuschel, A. and Feldmann, M. (2008) Therapist-assisted, Self-administered Bibliotherapy to Enhance Parental Competence: short- and long-term effects, *Behaviour Modification*, **32** (5), 659–81.

Hannigan, M. (1962) The Librarian in Bibliotherapy: pharmacist or bibliotherapist?, *Library Trends*, **11** (2), 184–98.

Hicks, D. (2006) *An Audit of Bibliotherapy/Books on Prescription Activity in England*, The Reading Agency.

Hynes, A. (1975) Bibliotherapy in the Circulating Library at Saint Elizabeth's Hospital, *Libri*, **25** (2), 144–8.

Jackson, E. P. (1962) Bibliotherapy and Reading Guidance: a tentative approach to theory, *Library Trends*, **11** (2), 118–26.

Johnson, R. S. (1998) Bibliotherapy: battling depression, *Library Journal*, **123** (10), 73–6.

Kenwright, M. (2010) Introducing and Supporting Written and Internet-based Guided CBT. In Bennett-Levy, J., Richards. D. A., Farrand, P., et al. (eds), *Oxford Guide to Low Intensity CBT Interventions*, Oxford University Press.

Kupshik, G. A. and Fisher, C. R. (1999) Assisted Bibliotherapy: effective, efficient treatment for moderate anxiety problems, *British Journal of General Practice*, **49** (1), 47–8.

Longden, E., Davis, P., Billington, J., Lampropoulou, S., Farrington, G., Magee, F., Walsh, E. and Corcoran, R. (2015) Shared Reading: assessing the intrinsic value of a literature-based health intervention, *Medical Humanities,* **41** (2),113–20.

McDaniel, W. B. (1956) Bibliotherapy – Some Historical and Contemporary Aspects, *ALA Bulletin,* **50**, 584–9.

Mains, J. A. and Scogin, F. (2003) The Effectiveness of Self-administered Treatments: a practice-friendly review of the research, *Journal of Clinical Psychology,* **59** (2), 237–46.

Mataix-Cols, D. and Marks, I. M. (2006) Self-help with Minimal Therapist Contact for Obsessive Compulsive Disorder: a review, *European Psychiatry,* **21** (2), 75–80.

Morley, C. (1919) *The Haunted Bookshop,* Dodo Press.

Morral, K. (2016) *Well into Words: an evaluation of the Kirklees Bibliotherapy Project,* http://media.wix.com/ugd/6b65c6_f430a267c13848bdbe55ae13aa52ecdf.pdf.

National Institute for Health and Care Excellence (2004a) *CG22 Anxiety: management of anxiety (panic disorder, with or without agoraphobia, and generalised anxiety disorder) in adults in primary, secondary and community care,* http://guidance.nice.org.uk/CG22.

National Institute for Health and Care Excellence (2004b) *CG23 Depression: management of depression in primary and secondary care (amended),* www.nice.org.uk/nicemedia/pdf/CG23NICEguidelineamended.pdf.

National Institute for Health and Care Excellence (2004c) *CG9 Eating disorders,* www.nice.org.uk/nicemedia/pdf/CG9FullGuideline.pdf.

National Institute for Health and Care Excellence (2009) *CG90 Depression: the treatment and management of depression in adults,* www.nice.org.uk/nicemedia/pdf/CG 90 QRG LR FINAL.pdf.

O'Sullivan, N., Davis, P., Billington J., Gonzalez-Diaz, V. and Corcoran, R. (2015) 'Shall I Compare Thee': the neural basis of literary awareness, and its benefits to cognition, *Cortex,* **73**, 144–57.

Pawson, R. (2006) *Evidence-based Policy: a realist perspective,* Sage.

Peterson Delaney, S. (1938) The Place of Bibliotherapy in a Hospital, *Library Journal,* **63**, 305–8.

Porter, A., Snooks, H., Lloyd, K., Peconi, J., Evans, A., and Russell, I. (2006) *An evaluation of Book Prescription Wales: final project report,* AWARD.

Porter, R. (2002) *Madness: a brief history,* Oxford University Press.

Reeves, T. and Stace, J. M. (2005) Improving Patient Access and Choice: assisted bibliography for mild to moderate stress/anxiety in primary care, *Journal of Psychiatric and Mental Health Nursing,* **12** (3), 341–6.

Richards, D. (2004) Self-help: empowering service users or aiding cash strapped mental health services?, *Journal of Mental Health,* **13** (2): 117–23.

Richardson, R., Richards, D. and Barkham, M. (2008) Self-help Books for People with Depression: a scoping review, *Journal of Mental Health*, **17** (5), 543–52.

Rosenblatt, L. M. (1938) *Literature as Exploration*, Heinemann.

Rubin, R. J. (1978a) *Bibliotherapy Sourcebook*, Oryx Press.

Rubin, R. J. (1978b) *Using Bibliotherapy: theory and practice*, Oryx Press.

Sclabassi, S. H. (1973) Literature as a Therapeutic Tool – review of the literature on bibliotherapy, *American Journal of Psychotherapy*, **27** (1), 70–77.

Shephard, B. (2002) *A War of Nerves: soldiers and psychiatrists, 1914–1994*, Pimlico.

Shorter, E. (1997) *A History of Psychiatry: from the era of the asylum to the age of Prozac*, Wiley.

Shrodes, C. (1949) *Bibliotherapy: a theoretical and clinical-experimental study*, University of California.

Tews, R. M. (1962) Introduction, *Library Trends*, **11** (2), 97–105.

The Reading Agency and BOP Consulting (2015) *Literature Review: the impact of reading for pleasure and empowerment*, https://readingagency.org.uk/news/The Impact of Reading for Pleasure and Empowerment.pdf.

The Reading Agency, Society of Chief Librarians and BOP Consulting (2016) *Reading Well Books on Prescription Evaluation 2015–16*, https://readingagency.org.uk/resources/1886.

Weimerskirch, P. (1965) Benjamin Rush and John Minson Galt II: pioneers of bibliotherapy, *Bulletin of the Medical Library Association*, **53** (4), 510–26.

White, J. (1995) Stresspac: a controlled trial of a self-help package for the anxiety disorders, *Behavioural and Cognitive Psychology*, **23** (2), 89–107.

White, J. (1998) 'Stresspac': three year follow up of a controlled trial of a self-help package for the anxiety disorders, *Behavioural and Cognitive Psychology*, **26** (1), 133–41.

Williams, C. and Martinez, R. (2008) Increasing access to CBT: stepped care and CBT models in practice, *Behavioural and Cognitive Psychology*, **36**, 675–83.

2

Theories of bibliotherapy

Sarah McNicol

Introduction

As discussed in Chapter 1, the aims of, and approaches to, bibliotherapy have changed over time. In the past, it was sometimes seen simply as a means of keeping patients content while therapies took place, but 21st-century bibliotherapy has much more ambitious aims: improving social and emotional wellbeing and increasing confidence and self-esteem. As such, some early theories attempting to explain the positive results of bibliotherapy now appear simplistic: for example, encouraging patients with depression to read books with 'amusing anecdotes or . . . jovial comradeship' (McAlister, 1950, 356).

As the case studies in Part 2 illustrate, bibliotherapy activities that currently take place across many settings and with a range of target audiences report significant impacts on the quality of life of participants. But while much attention has been paid to demonstrating the effectiveness of bibliotherapy, finding out *how* it works has proved more challenging. A typical example is a study into the use of bibliotherapy to treat adolescent depression (Ackerson et al., 1998). Here, the researchers used a number of standardized psychological instruments to compare a treatment group who took part in an intervention with a control group who did not. Based upon statistical analysis of subjects' scores on these tests, the study concluded 'bibliotherapy may be an effective treatment for adolescents experiencing depressive symptoms'. The readers' responses to the book, however, were ignored and nowhere in the study were the readers' reactions to the book or its content described (Dysart-Gale, 2007).

This chapter outlines some of the theories behind bibliotherapy and demonstrates how they relate to practical bibliotherapy initiatives found in library settings. This includes schemes focused on the individual, such as

Books on Prescription, as well as collective activities such as shared reading, and those concerned with the consumption of literature, such as reading groups, as well as those focused on its creation – for example, creative writing groups. Practical examples from the case studies presented in this book are used to illustrate the theories described, along with findings from a study of health comics readers (McNicol 2015; 2017). However, before focusing on bibliotherapy specifically, it is useful to consider the notion of reading 'stances' more generally.

Reading stances

Louise Rosenblatt (1994) describes reading as having two stances, *efferent* and *aesthetic*, positioned at each end of a continuum. A stance defines the ways in which readers interact with a text and reflects their purpose for reading and their attitudes towards, and expectations of, a particular text. An efferent stance signifies a factual perspective, while an aesthetic stance represents a more emotional focus. As they engage with a text, readers are constantly making meaning using both stances and, although they may make greater use of one than of the other, they often adopt multiple stances during the reading of a single text. Typically, an efferent stance involves a more literal reading, with the goal of extracting information. An efferent reading can be thought of as factual, analytical and cognitive. A reader who is reading primarily from an efferent stance directs their attention outward, focusing on the knowledge they expect to take from the reading event. The reader concentrates on 'the information, the concepts, the guides to action' (Rosenblatt, 1994, 27) that are contained within the text in order to create public, rather than private, meanings. The aesthetic stance, on the other hand, is a more emotional reading and frequently focuses on the personal journey a reader takes during the act of reading. An aesthetic stance is characterized by a reader focusing on their immediate participation in the reading event as he or she 'participates in the tensions, conflicts, and resolutions of the images, ideas, and scenes as they unfold' (Rosenblatt, 2006, 1067). This involves a 'distancing from ''reality''' (Rosenblatt, 1994, 31) when the reader focuses their attention on the 'associations, feelings, attitudes and ideas' (Rosenblatt, 1994, 25) that are aroused by the text and 'savors the qualities of the feelings, ideas, situations, scenes, personalities, and emotions that are called forth' (Rosenblatt, 2006, 1373) to create their own, private, meanings. Texts do offer clues to the reader about what stance to adopt; for instance, it is usual to expect that a poem will be read from an aesthetic stance and a car repair manual from an efferent one. However, stance is not tied exclusively to particular kinds of texts. In other words, a reader can choose to read any given text aesthetically, efferently or using a combination of both approaches. For example, a reader may read a novel in one way for pleasure reading and in a very different way if they are being examined on the same novel as part of a literature course.

Within bibliotherapy, a text may be read efferently, for example to gain factual information about a health condition or to assist with decision-making. This approach is commonly found in CBT-based approaches such as Books on Prescription schemes. In contrast, the aesthetic stance is more usually associated with creative forms of bibliotherapy that emphasize the importance of the reading experience, focusing on imaginative and personal responses to texts. For example, fables and fairy tales are commonly used in this type of bibliotherapy because they provide a degree of disassociation while still allowing the reader to relate their problems and experiences to characters in the stories.

Cognitive-Behavioural Therapy models

To consider the first of these contrasting approaches: many bibliotherapy schemes, especially those associated with clinical bibliotherapy, adopt an approach based on Cognitive-Behavioural Therapy (CBT). For example, the UK National Institute for Health and Care Excellence (NICE) has produced guidelines recommending the effectiveness of self-based help based on CBT principles for a range of conditions, including anxiety (CG113), depression (CG90) and common mental health disorders (CG123).

In broad terms, CBT is a way of talking about how you think about yourself, the world and other people, and how what you do affects your thoughts and feelings. CBT is based on the concept that thoughts, feelings, physical sensations and actions are interconnected, and that negative thoughts and feelings can trap people in a vicious cycle. It helps to break problems down into smaller parts and change negative patterns. CBT deals with current problems rather than issues from the past and looks for practical ways to improve a patient's state of mind on a daily basis (National Health Service, 2016). Bibliotherapy based on a CBT model typically relies on self-help books which work to 'correct' negative behaviours by offering alternative, positive actions. For example, many of the titles offered through Books on Prescription schemes (Frude, 2005) can be thought of as a form of CBT. Books on Prescription resources provide information on mental health problems such as depression, anxiety and sleep problems. As well as providing information, many of the books offer techniques and strategies for successfully managing and overcoming mental health problems. These self-help books often offer step-by-step treatment programmes with exercises, self-assessments and diary sheets. A number of authors talk about the importance of structure in change (e.g. Bohart and Tallman, 1999; Lambert and Ogles, 2004) and the step-by-step approaches provided by these resources afford this type of structure.

Some titles in Books on Prescription schemes present self-help versions of the kind of therapy that might be given by a professional, but as Floyd (2003) suggests, self-help books could enhance self-efficacy: when patients see progress, they are able to attribute some of this progress to their own efforts, rather than the efforts of their counsellors. However, it is important to remember that, in most cases, there is no discussion element to this model of bibliotherapy; the patient undertakes the exercises alone and does not usually discuss their reading with a healthcare or other professional as part of the process. (See Chapter 1 for an overview of the development of Books on Prescription).

Fiction reading and transportation

While bibliotherapy schemes focused on self-help materials, such as Books on Prescription, are largely based on CBT approaches, other forms of bibliotherapy, especially those making use of fiction or poetry, are more usually based on theories associated with reader development and the reading experience.

To put bibliotherapy initiatives in context, it is important to remember that research suggests that reading for pleasure generally is effective in tackling common mental issues such as anxiety and stress and in raising awareness about health issues (BOP Consulting, 2015). For example, in an online poll, people who regularly read for pleasure reported fewer feelings of stress and depression than non-readers and stronger feelings of relaxation were associated with reading than with television or technology activities. Regular readers also reported higher levels of self-esteem, better sleep patterns and a greater ability to cope with difficult situations (Billington 2015). Large-scale studies in the USA have even shown that engaging in reading, especially fiction reading, is associated with a subsequent lower risk of dementia (BOP Consulting, 2015).

A key element in understanding the potential impact of reading is the idea of a 'transportation effect' (Green, 2008). Along with related terms such as 'absorption' (Slater and Rouner, 2002), 'escapism' (Brewster, 2016) and 'involvement' (Moyer-Gusé, 2008), this suggests that stories have the power to make readers feel transported into the world of the narrative and even participate in the action as one of the characters. Transportation has been defined as 'an integrative melding of attention, imagery and feelings, focused on story events' (Green, 2006). In some studies, transportation is measured using a self-report scale with statements such as 'I was emotionally involved in the narrative while reading it' and 'I could picture myself in the scene of the events described in the narrative' (Green, 2006).

This process of transportation offers a chance to experiment with different types of roles (Booth, 1988) and to explore what it would be like to be someone else (Palmer, 1992). Schrank and Engels (1981) refer to an 'affiliation' between the reader and character as a type of therapeutic transference relationship. In this way, characters in stories may serve as role models, especially when a reader can more easily connect their own lives and experiences to those of a protagonist. A reader may connect themselves with the story in a number of ways, most obviously through being reminded of their own experiences through reading a description of a similar event happening to a character. In such instances, characters can illustrate the costs and benefits of different courses of action or can provide reassurance that the reader is not alone in the issues they are facing. It is argued that 'transportation into a narrative world can lead to real-world belief (and behaviour) change' (Green, 2006). Green describes three ways in which transportation can affect readers: creating connection with characters; reducing counterarguments; and making narrative events seem more like real experiences.

When a reader likes, or identifies particularly strongly with, a character, the implications of events experienced or assertions made by that character may carry greater weight, perhaps even leading the reader to seek to emulate the actions of admired characters. Furthermore, it has been argued that the more similar to them a character is, the more a reader will identify with that character (Green, 2006). Whilst similarities based simply on demographic characteristics such as age, race and gender can be important, similarity between the reader's story and that of the character may, in fact, lead to a much stronger sense of transportation. In addition to identifying with a character, a reader can project their own emotions or interpretations within the fictional context. Characters with whom a reader identifies may offer templates for 'possible selves' (Markus and Nurius, 1986). Literature offers a safe space to experiment with alternatives as, while reading invites participation, it also allows the reader a degree of emotional distance and control, since they may remove themselves from the experience at any time. As Oatley (1999) suggests, narratives provide a middle ground where emotions can be experienced sufficiently for their meaning to be understood, but not so greatly that they are overwhelming.

Whilst the theory of transportation clearly has importance for bibliotherapy schemes that make use of fiction, there are also theories that specifically seek to explain the impact of bibliotherapy. These are most commonly based on psychological or counselling theories.

Identification, catharsis and insight

A common approach is to consider bibliotherapy as a three-stage process:

1 identification and projection
2 abreaction and catharsis
3 insight and integration.

Based on psychological approaches to storytelling and drawing on counselling theory, this approach underpins bibliotherapy in both clinical and community settings (e.g. Morawski, 1997; Shrodes, 1955). Identification is an empathetic response that occurs when a reader associates themselves with a character or situation in a literary work. They examine the behaviours and motives of characters and start to explore their own perceptions and actions, for example, recalling related incidents from their own life. For instance, in a study in which interviewees were asked to read a number of health-related comics about a condition they, or a family member, suffered from (McNicol, 2015), a typical reaction demonstrating identification with the story was:

> they're like real life stories almost . . . it's good 'cos it's almost a story about what's going on with it, so you can sort of relate to it.

Further examples of identification are offered in Chapter 6, where Fiona Bailey discusses how participants relate John Clare's poem 'I Am' to their own experiences of stigma and creativity. This identification can lead to imaginary role-play or simulation as the reader puts themselves in the position of the character.

The second stage, catharsis, is when the reader shares many of the same thoughts and feelings as the characters in the story and may address feelings associated with the incidents from their own life which they recalled during the identification stage. Readers may express intense emotions through the fictional character; Fuhriman, Barlow and Wanless (1989) describe a 'vicarious cleansing' as the reader releases emotional energy through fictional characters. In an example of catharsis from the study of comics readers mentioned above (McNicol, 2015), a reader goes a stage further from simple identification and realizes she shares experiences and feelings with characters in the text; they remind her of the conversations she had with her mother when she was younger, and the frustration she felt:

> . . . you've got this kid going on about what they want to do and then her reply [and a thought bubble showing] what she's actually thinking. And I think that reply there is exactly what my mum used to say. It's spot on to when we used to ask things, she'd say, 'Oh, I'll just see how I'm feeling' and you think, 'How are we going to know? . . . It's so annoying, so frustrating'.

In Chapter 9 Cristina Deberti Martins offers further compelling examples of the process of catharsis when relating patients' reactions to a poem.

The final stage, insight, is when the reader realizes that they relate to the character or situation and learn to deal more effectively with their own personal issues. Thus, they begin to approach a problem on a more intellectual level in order to 'come to a better understanding of [their] own motivations or achieve an awareness of something applicable to [their] own life' (Hoaglund, 1972, 391). They begin to understand the reasons behind their behaviours and attitudes and may even develop communication skills allowing them to verbalize their feelings through modelling fictional characters (Fuhriman, Barlow and Wanless, 1989). In the comics study (McNicol, 2015), insight occurred when the act of reading prompted interviewees to reflect on their own actions and the ways in which they were dealing with their (or their relative's) health condition, for example:

> The narrative about people nagging her and being a bit overprotective and . . . almost thinking they knew best made me think, 'Maybe I shouldn't . . . Maybe I should be slightly more . . .'. I don't think I'm not understanding, but just . . . appreciate how hard it must be a bit more . . .'

Arleen Hynes and Mary Hynes-Berry (2012) have further developed this identification–catharsis–insight model to describe a four-step biblio-therapeutic process. The first of these steps is recognition: the reader's attention is caught as they recognize an understanding of a person or experience. This recognition might happen spontaneously, or following probing by a facilitator or remarks from other participants in a group setting. Furthermore, recognition does not necessarily relate to a specific piece of literature, but could apply to a pattern of responses, for instance, if a participant experiences similar reactions to a number of pieces of literature over a series of sessions. Rather than viewing catharsis as a separate stage, Hynes and Hynes-Berry (2012) describe this phenomenon as a profound experience of recognition that can occur when a reader identifies with something in the text deeply or when the literature touches buried memories or emotions.

The second step of this process is 'examination' as the reader examines issues and asks questions about their response to them. This leads to the third stage of 'juxtaposition' as a deeper level of understanding is reached and the reader considers their initial understanding in light of new feelings and ideas exposed by the 'examination' process. Comparing their original values, concepts, attitudes or feelings to those after the examination stage can lead to four possible options: affirmation of their original position; modification of this position; recognition that the first idea was, in fact, not valid; or uncertainty. In this way, Hynes and Hynes-Berry (2012) argue, literature can correct discrepancies as a reader comes to realize that their opinion was based on an incorrect understanding. Literature can offer role models or suggest alternative options, but based on patterns of response rather than exact mirroring of a situation.

The final stage is 'self-application', as the reader evaluates their impressions and insights, and integrates them into their inner self. Evaluation represents a new level of recognition and examination, as the reader considers how their attitudes and behaviours are affected by new viewpoints. Self-application occurs as the reader identifies or 'names' (Percy, 1975) a description found in a work of literature, but filters it for their own life or situation. Thus, 'the whole process culminates in a new, deeply personal meaning that will inform future attitudes and actions' (Hynes and Hynes-Berry, 2012, 31). It is important to emphasize that the insight produced may either reinforce existing beliefs or behaviours or, alternatively, may create a new solution.

According to Hynes and Hynes-Berry, these four steps are always followed in the same sequence, but not at uniform rate, and frequently not during a single session. Language is key, both as a stimulus and an agent in the process. The authors also stress the importance of discussion and the need to distinguish between processes that involve facilitated discussion and those that involve merely prescribing books.

The interaction of text and reader

While these broad models of the ways in bibliotherapy can work are helpful, it is important to remember that bibliotherapy may not work in the same way, or to the same extent, for all readers. Systematic reviews synthesizing the results of randomized control trials (RCTs) have found that bibliotherapy is most effective when used with volunteers rather than a wider cross-section of the population (Fanner and Urquhart, 2008). This increased success with those who volunteer to undergo treatment, rather than those who are referred to it by medical professionals, suggests that personal motivation may have an impact on the effectiveness of bibliotherapy interventions (Brewster, Sen and Cox, 2012).

The types of 'reader attributes' that may impact substantially on the outcomes of a reading experience include the reader's level of need for emotional support; their attitude towards their condition; their self-perception; their need for information; their attitudes towards the texts; and demographic characteristics such as age and gender (McNicol, 2017). Naturally, some of these factors might be of greater relevance for certain individuals. The interaction of these factors with attributes of particular texts, such as narrative and characterization, can produce a number of effects, including resonance, reassurance, empathy, confirmation, companionship, positive effects on mood and increased awareness of alternative perspectives.

Restitution, chaos and quest narratives

Just as not all readers will react in the same way to a particular literary work, not all texts are written to produce the same type of response. Arthur Frank (2013, 187) outlined three patterns of illness narrative or 'imaginative conceptions of illness': the 'restitution' narrative portrays illness as a temporary condition where the aim is to recover from disease and return to a previous state of health and normality; the 'chaos' narrative imagines life never getting better; and finally the 'quest' narrative focuses on learning and on spiritual and psychological transformation rather than physical outcomes. (See Chapter 3 for a more detailed description of Frank's work). In the study of health comics referred to previously (McNicol, 2015), it was interesting to note how strongly a number of interviewees rejected texts which they interpreted as presenting restitution or chaos narratives. The simplistic premise of the restitution narrative was dismissed as highly unsatisfying, for example:

> It's a bit limiting . . . it would be like the equivalent of someone saying, 'It'll all work out fine in the end' . . . 'Pull yourself together', 'Always darkest before dawn'. Maybe it's a little trite . . .

Equally, the confusing and pessimistic nature of chaos narratives was found to be unsettling and unhelpful:

> One of them was terrifying . . . a bit freaky . . . somebody's mind that's gone a bit crazy, isn't it? . . . this one's a bit doom and gloom, you'd think, 'Oh crikey' . . .

Much better received were narratives describing how to accept, live with and better understand health conditions or, as Frank (2013, 117) says, stories that 'tell of searching for alternative ways of being ill':

> It just brought it back to my awareness because I live with it all the time I don't even think about it . . . it brought things up into my mind that were in my mind but . . . suppressed . . . I try to think that I haven't got it, so I was like, 'I have got it and this is what I've got to deal with'. It made me realise that I'm doing alright considering . . .   (Quoted in McNicol, 2015).

These quotes demonstrate Frank's (2003 187) argument that, 'the stories that people hear shape the stories they tell about themselves'. Individuals may react in different ways to different narratives and this can have a significant impact on the ways in which they think about their lives and their health.

Community models of bibliotherapy

Bibliotherapy has been described as is 'a very individual exploration of the self' (Brewster, 2007, 15) and, thus far, this chapter has focused on the bibliotherapy experiences for an individual reader. Approaches termed 'reading bibliotherapy' see healing as taking place through the act of reading itself and an individual reader's response to a text. Books on Prescription and similar schemes offering lists of suggested texts can be described as examples of reading bibliotherapy. The key interaction takes place between the text and the reader; the person who made the book suggestion is unlikely to have a role in the therapeutic process. However, as the case studies presented in Part 2 illustrate, community support or peer support is an important aspect of many bibliotherapy initiatives. Interactive or community bibliotherapy places less emphasis on the act of reading and more on guided dialogue with the material. For example, in Hynes and Hynes-Berry's (2012) four-step process described above, recognition often occurs as a result of the discussion around literature, as much as from the literature itself.

This process of discussion is central to many schemes developed in recent years, such as Shared Reading, but it has been also been used as part of self-based help models. For example, East Renfrewshire Council's Health Access (Cather, 2007) is based on a Books on Prescription model with a similar range of self-help books, but also has Health Information Points in libraries staffed by health professionals. Training is given to library staff so that they can perform a 'health reference interview' which builds on the librarian's traditional reference interview and encourages librarians to become 'information counsellors' and collaborate with other professionals.

Whilst the key interaction in the East Renfrewshire scheme is between librarian and reader, there are also models of community bibliotherapy that adopt a peer-support approach, for instance reading aloud and book groups where literature is taken away to read individually and then discussed in a group meeting. But whichever model was used, Brewster (2016) found that three interacting elements were vital to the implementation of successful groups: the group environment, the group facilitator and the literature itself.

Group bibliotherapy has a number of potential advantages. Perhaps the most significant is that important experiences or insights may be possible through interaction not just with the facilitator, but with other group members too. As described in the case study of psychiatric patients in Chapter 8, participants become aware that their feelings are shared by others in the group. As Rosenblatt wrote:

> As we exchange experiences, we point to those elements of the text that best illustrate or support our interpretations. We may help one another to attend to words, phrases, images, scenes, that we have overlooked or slighted. We may be led to reread the text and revise our own interpretation. Sometimes we may be strengthened in our own sense of having 'done justice to' the text, without denying its potentialities for other interpretations. Sometimes the give-and-take may lead to a general increase in insight and even to a consensus.
>
> (Rosenblatt, 1994, 146)

A study of peer-led recovery groups based around a self-help workbook for people with eating disorders demonstrated that sharing of lived experiences can improve self-esteem, self-efficacy and social support (Fukui et al., 2010). The fact that potential differences between group members were less marked than those between the patient and a professional was felt to be critical, as was the fact that people were able to draw on lived experiences in their responses rather than theoretical principles.

Furthermore, as several studies examining readability have found, a high level of literacy is often required to read CBT-based self-help books (Martinez et al., 2008; Richardson, Richards and Barkham, 2010). Group bibliotherapy may therefore be helpful for those with lower literacy levels, lower confidence in their literacy skills or a reduced ability to concentrate due to their condition. They can access texts through reading aloud and discussion that would not be accessible to them otherwise.

Shared Reading

One of the schemes specifically targeted towards these groups who may find traditional forms of bibliotherapy less accessible is Shared Reading.[1] Importantly, in contrast to some self-help-based forms of bibliotherapy, schemes such as Shared Reading do not expect to find simple literal answers or comfortable solutions to perceived problems. This type of bibliotherapy has different aims, being focused on the value of deep mental involvement and seeking meaning in a broad sense. An assessment of the cultural value of this scheme identified five intrinsic elements of the experience that help to explain the theory underpinning the model. The first is liveliness: in contrast to many other reading groups, the texts in a Shared Reading group are read aloud rather than being read in advance. This model has been described as 'a form of immediate *doing*, rather than solitary interpretation in measured retrospect' (Longden et al., 2015, 10; emphasis in original). There is, therefore, an element of unpredictability as group members respond to the texts in a very immediate way. The second element is 'creative inarticulacy': in contrast to self-help books in which the procedure is top-down in terms of the naming of procedures, treatments and so forth, in this model, language tends to be much more uncertain and tentative as group members try to find ways of expressing emergent ideas. The third element of Shared Reading is the importance of the emotional: demonstrating the 'use' of literature, but in an affective, rather than an instrumental, sense. The fourth element is the ways in which literature can prompt personal stories, or 'self-disclosing talk' (Longden et al., 2015, 20). Although the text is fictional, it can feel immediately very real when read aloud, prompting participants to shift from outward attention to inward attention as they review their own experiences in the light of the literary context. The final element is the group itself: in particular, similarities and differences in their responses to the text.

Creative writing and bibliotherapy

While the main focus of this chapter has been on the reading of published texts, in line with the majority of library-based bibliotherapy schemes, it is also important to consider approaches to bibliotherapy that support writing activities. Based on the idea that writing about traumatic or emotional events can lead to improved health, many creative writing approaches draw on the notion of expressive writing pioneered by James Pennebaker in the 1980s (Pennebaker and Beall, 1986). This typically involves responding to a 'task' to write about a traumatic event or experience for 20 minutes on three or four consecutive days. Numerous trials have claimed benefits for this approach that include shorter hospital stays (Solano et al., 2007), fewer health visits (Baikie, 2008), improved immunity (Pennebaker, Kiecolt-Glaser and Glaser, 1988) and reduced anxiety and depression (Graf, Gaudiano and Geller, 2008).

Pennebaker explains the benefits of expressive writing in terms of both an 'inhibition theory' and a 'cognitive change theory'. Inhibition theory states that writing helps to disclose thoughts and feelings that would otherwise remain inhibited, while his 'cognitive change theory' suggests that writing helps people to 'reorganize' their thoughts and feelings about traumatic experiences, thus creating 'coherence' and/or 'story' and 'meaning' (Pennebaker and Seagal, 1999).

Other approaches to creative writing adopt a more fluid approach: rather than setting a writing 'task', each individual is encouraged to progress at their own pace and in their own way. A writer may be encouraged to set out their feelings on the page initially, then move on to begin to shape and redraft their story, perhaps fictionalizing or retelling the initial story from a different point of view. Significant insights and understandings are gained at each stage as the writer reflects and becomes a reader of their story, as well as its author.

A possible framework for understanding ways in which writing can help us to achieve shifts towards self-understanding, coherence and meaning is suggested by recent work in neurophysiology and cognitive science which suggest that developmental creative writing may enable us to reconnect with more 'felt, bodily' aspects of our self-experience (Damasio, 2000). Nicholls (2009) argues that expressive writing might be seen as enabling participants to begin connecting with felt experiences (emotions, traumatic memories and so forth). Release occurs not merely as a result of 'disclosing' difficult experiences, but by connecting with how the writer feels about an experience, rather than what they think about the experience (or think that they should feel about it). As with reading, it is argued that writing a narrative can give individuals a degree of distance from their illness, allowing them to better cope with the emotions involved (Carlick and Biley, 2004).

Conclusion

It is important to point out that the theories described in this chapter represent just some of the more common approaches to bibliotherapy, particularly those found within a library or other non-clinical setting. Other researchers from medical fields have adopted theories more closely based on psychoanalytic perspectives such as the use of the psychoanalytical 'frame' described by Cristina Deberti Martins in Chapter 9.

In outlining different theories and approaches to bibliotherapy, this chapter does not attempt to suggest that one model is superior to another. Each approach may be suited to different individuals or at different times in an individual's life: whilst some people may respond well to CBT-based methods, others will gain more from fiction reading and community models of bibliotherapy. Perhaps the key concept linking all forms of bibliotherapy is Rosenblatt's statement that 'Literature provides a *living-through*, not simply *knowledge about*' (Rosenblatt, 1968, 38; emphasis in original). The theories described in this chapter all consider the ways in which texts can connect with lived experiences, whether in a very direct and immediate sense, as in the case of CBT-based approaches, or in more abstract and indirect ways, through the process of transportation for example. Whichever model of bibliotherapy is adopted, however, it is important for those managing the activities to develop an understanding of theories underpinning the intervention. It is only through doing so that they can make decisions about which models of bibliotherapy may be most effective for a given setting and audience, as well as appropriate ways to select texts, lead discussions, provide support and so forth. We do not simply need to know whether bibliotherapy works; to be effective practitioners, we also need to appreciate how and why a particular model works in order to ensure we meet the needs of different individuals and communities who may benefit from interventions.

Notes

1 www.thereader.org.uk/about/whatwedo/#whatissr.

References

Ackerson, J., Scogin, F., McKendree-Smith, N. and Lyman, R. D. (1998) Cognitive Bibliotherapy for Mild and Moderate Adolescent Depressive Symptomatology, *Journal of Consulting and Clinical Psychology*, **66** (4), 685–90.

Baikie, K. A. (2008) Who Does Expressive Writing Work For? Examination of alexithymia, splitting, and repressive coping style as moderators of the expressive writing paradigm, *British Journal of Health Psychology*, **13** (1), 61–6.

Billington, J. (2015) *Reading between the Lines: the benefits of reading for pleasure*, Quick Reads, http://manuscritdepot.com/documentspdf/Galaxy-Quick-Reads-Report-FINAL%20.pdf.

Bohart, A. and Tallman, K. (1999) *How Clients Make Therapy Work: the process of active self-healing*, American Psychological Association.

Booth, W. (1988) *The Company We Keep, an Ethics of Fiction*, University of California Press.

BOP Consulting (2015) *Literature Review: the impact of reading for pleasure and empowerment*, The Reading Agency and BOP Consulting, https://readingagency.org.uk/news/The%20Impact%20of%20Reading%20for%20Pleasure%20and%20Empowerment.pdf.

Brewster, L. (2007) (Brewster, E. A.) *'Medicine for the Soul': bibliotherapy and the public library*, MA thesis, University of Sheffield, http://dagda.shef.ac.uk/dispub/dissertations/2006-07/External/Brewster_Elizabeth_MALib.pdf.

Brewster, L. (2016) More Benefit from a Well-stocked Library than a Well-stocked Pharmacy: how do readers use books as therapy? In Rothbauer, P. M., Skjerdingstad, K. I., McKechnie, L. E. F. and Oterholm, K. (eds), *Plotting the Reading Experience: theory/policy/politics*, Wilfred Laurier University Press.

Brewster, L., Sen, B. and Cox, A. (2012) Legitimising Bibliotherapy: evidence-based discourses in health care, *Journal of Documentation*, **68** (2), 185–205.

Carlick, A. and Biley, F. C. (2004) Thoughts on the Therapeutic Use of Narrative in the Promotion of Coping in Cancer Care, *European Journal of Cancer Care*, **13** (4), 308–17.

Cather, C. (2007) *To Every Reader Her Book: creating bibliotherapy for women*, www.shinelib.org.uk/assets/0000/0294/To_Every_Reader_Her_Book_MSc_Dissertation_By_Christine_Catherpdf.pdf

Damasio, A. (2000) *The Feeling of What Happens*, Harvest Books.

Dysart-Gale, D. (2007) Lost in Translation: bibliotherapy and evidence-based medicine, *Journal of Medical Humanities*, **29** (1), 33–43.

Fanner, D. and Urquhart, C. (2008) Bibliotherapy for Mental Health Service Users. Part 1: a systematic review, *Health Information and Libraries Journal*, **25** (4), 237–52.

Floyd, M. R. (2003) Bibliotherapy as an Adjunct to Psychotherapy for Depression in Older Adults, *Journal of Clinical Psychology*, **59** (2), 187–95.

Frank, A. W. (2013) *The Wounded Storyteller: body, illness and ethics*, 2nd edn, University of Chicago Press.

Frude, N. (2005) Book Prescriptions — a strategy for delivering psychological treatment in the primary care setting, *Mental Health Review Journal*, **10** (4), 30–3.

Fuhriman, A., Barlow, S. and Wanless, J. (1989) Words, Imagination, Meaning: towards change, *Psychotherapy*, **26** (2), 149–56.

Fukui, S., Davidson, L., Holter, M. and Rapp, C. (2010) Pathways to Recovery (PTR): impact of peer-led group participation on mental health recovery outcomes, *Psychiatric Rehabilitation Journal*, **34** (1), 42–8.

Graf, M. C., Gaudiano, B. A. and Geller, P. A. (2008) Written Emotional Disclosure: a controlled study of the benefits of expressive writing homework in outpatient psychotherapy, *Psychotherapy Research*, **18** (4), 389–99.

Green, M. C. (2006) Narratives and Cancer Communication, *Journal of Communication*, **56** (Supplement s1), S163–83.

Green, M. C. (2008) Research Challenges in Narrative Persuasion, *Information Design Journal*, **16** (1), 47–52.

Hoaglund, J. (1972) Bibliotherapy: aiding children in personality development, *Elementary English* **49** (3), 390–94.

Hynes, A. M. and Hynes-Berry, M. (2012) Biblio/Poetry Therapy – the Interactive Process: a handbook, North Star.

Lambert, J. J. and Ogles, B. M. (2004) The Efficacy and Effectiveness of Psychotherapy. In Lambert, M. J. (ed), *Bergin and Garfield's Handbook of Psychotherapy and Behavior Change*, 5th edn, Wiley.

Longden, E., Davis, P., Billington, J., Lampropoulou, S., Farrington, G., Magee, F., Walsh E. and Corcoran, R. (2015) Cultural Value: assessing the intrinsic value of The Reader Organization's Shared Reading Scheme, www.thereader.org.uk/wp-content/uploads/2017/06/Cultural-Value.pdf.

McAlister, C. (1950) Bibliotherapy, *American Journal of Nursing*, **50** (6), 356–57.

McNicol, S. (2015) *The Impact of Educational Comics on Feelings and Attitudes Towards Health Conditions: interviews with patients and family members*, https://doi.org/10.6084/m9.figshare.1512330.v1.

McNicol, S. (2017) The Potential of Educational Comics as a Health Information Medium, *Health Information and Libraries Journal*, **34** (1), 20–31.

Markus, H. and Nurius, P. (1986) Possible Selves, *American Psychologist*, **41** (9), 954–69.

Martinez, R., Whitfield, G., Dafters, R. and Williams, C. (2008) Can People Read Self-help Manuals for Depression? A challenge for the stepped care model and book prescription schemes, *Behavioural and Cognitive Psychology*, **36** (1), 89–97.

Morawski, C. (1997) A Role for Bibliotherapy in Teacher Education, *Reading Horizons*, **37** (3), 243–58.

Moyer-Gusé, E. (2008) Toward a Theory of Entertainment Persuasion: explaining the persuasive effects of entertainment-education messages, *Communication Theory*, **18** (3), 407–25.

National Health Service (2016) *Cognitive Behavioural Therapy (CBT)*, www.nhs.uk/conditions/Cognitive-behavioural-therapy/Pages/Introduction.aspx

Nicholls, S. (2009) Beyond Expressive Writing: evolving models of developmental creative writing, *Journal of Health Psychology*, **14** (2), 171–180.

Oatley, K. (1999) Why Fiction may be Twice as True as Fact: fiction as cognitive and emotional simulation, *Review of General Psychology*, **3** (2), 101–17.

Palmer, F. (1992) *Literature and Moral Understanding. a philosophical essay on ethics, aesthetics, education, and culture*, Clarendon Press.

Pennebaker, J. W. and Beall, S. K. (1986) Confronting a Traumatic Event: toward an understanding of inhibition and disease, *Journal of Abnormal Psychology*, **95** (3), 274–81.

Pennebaker, J. W. and Seagal, J. D. (1999) Forming a Story: the health benefits of narrative, *Journal of Clinical Psychology*, **55** (10), 1243–54.

Pennebaker, J. W., Kiecolt-Glaser, J. K. and Glaser, R. (1988) Disclosure of Traumas and Immune Function: health implications for psychotherapy, *Journal of Consulting and Clinical Psychology*, **56** (2), 239–45.

Percy, W. (1975) *Message in a Bottle*, Farrar, Strauss and Giroux.

Richardson, R., Richards, D. and Barkham, M. (2010) Self-help Books for People with Depression: the role of the therapeutic relationship, *Behavioural and Cognitive Psychology*, **38** (1), 67–81.

Rosenblatt, L. M. (1968) *Literature as Exploration*, Noble and Noble.

Rosenblatt, L. M. (1994) *The Reader, the Text, the Poem: the transactional theory of the literary work*, Southern Illinois University Press.

Rosenblatt, L. M. (2006) The Transactional Theory of Reading and Writing. In Ruddell, R. B. and Unrau, N. J. (eds), *Theoretical Models and Processes of Reading*, 5th edn, International Reading Association.

Schrank, F. A. and Engels, D. W. (1981) Bibliotherapy as a Counselling Adjunct: research findings, *Personnel and Guidance Journal*, **60** (3), 143–7.

Shrodes, C. (1955) Bibliotherapy, *The Reading Teacher*, **9**, 24–30.

Slater, M. D. and Rouner, D. (2002) Entertainment-education and Elaboration Likelihood: understanding the processing of narrative persuasion, *Communication Theory*, **12** (2), 173–91.

Solano, L., Pepe, L., Donati, V., Persichetti, S., Laudani, G. and Colaci, A. (2007) Differential Health Effects of Written Processing of the Experience of a Surgical Operation in High and Low Risk Conditions, *Journal of Clinical Psychology*, **63** (4), 357–69.

3

Bibliotherapy, illness narratives and narrative medicine

Liz Brewster

Introduction

Humans are said to be natural storytellers. Narrative brings a structure to communication that helps to make sense of the world around us. The recognition of the importance of stories and the use of narrative can be seen in many aspects of bibliotherapy, which may recommend the reading of fictional and autobiographical narratives to gain insight and improve mental health and wellbeing. But it is not only mental health that can benefit. Patients with physical illnesses may find meaning and understanding in reading autobiographical accounts of others who have undergone and articulated similar experiences to them. Illness narratives and narrative medicine are well theorized within the sociological and clinical literature, but have rarely been examined in relation to the use of bibliotherapy in practice. Looking at illness narratives and the theories around them may help to expand understandings of bibliotherapy by identifying how other texts may be used to benefit to health and wellbeing.

Stories can also be used to help medical professionals to understand the illness experience from a patient perspective. In medicine, narrative forms the core of the interaction between a clinician and a patient, telling the story of an illness and, in some cases, its resolution. Narrative medicine uses these patient stories, or stories written by clinicians about their experiences with patients and their treatment, to engage audiences including other patients and clinicians (Greenhalgh and Hurwitz, 1999). This narrative medicine can be seen as a form of bibliotherapy in clinical practice, increasing understanding and knowledge about a particular mental or physical health condition and helping to increase communication.

This chapter brings together research on bibliotherapy with medical sociology on illness narratives and narrative medicine. It explores the different forms this relationship between illness narratives, narrative medicine and bibliotherapy may take. It draws on previous research on illness narratives and narrative medicine and contrasts it with current models of bibliotherapy to conclude that the potential use of stories about health, illness and medicine stretch beyond current practice. It suggests some areas where connections between illness narratives, narrative medicine and bibliotherapy may be further explored.

Bibliotherapy: purposes and practices

Bibliotherapy is well established as the use of written materials to improve mental health and wellbeing, but questions remain around what type of books it is most useful to recommend (Brewster, 2009). There are two main models of bibliotherapy. First, bibliotherapy using books that contain structured education and provide information and support around diagnosed conditions such as depression and anxiety (Chamberlain, Heaps and Robert, 2008). Often using cognitive-behavioural therapeutic techniques, this form of bibliotherapy is currently delivered in UK public libraries via the Reading Well Books on Prescription scheme (The Reading Agency, 2015). The focus is on self-help and improving symptoms of mental health problems.

Second, there is bibliotherapy using imaginative literature such as novels, poetry and short stories (Billington et al., 2010). This form of bibliotherapy is sometimes delivered in group reading models, where imaginative literature is discussed and related to life events (Dowrick et al., 2012). While the focus is not directly on mental health and wellbeing, participants often report they experience improved wellbeing and increased understanding of life events. A sense of connection and recognition from seeing experiences represented on the page has been identified as a beneficial outcome (Brewster, 2016). Also associated with reading imaginative literature are the phenomena of the enjoyment of getting swept up in a story and being distracted from life events as a form of escapism (Brewster, 2016). As well as schemes that deliver this form of bibliotherapy in group settings, individuals also identify benefits in finding books for themselves and reading them independently (Brewster, 2016).

Regardless of whether self-help or imaginative literature titles are recommended, bibliotherapy has several purposes. It can provide a perspective on a topic not previously considered. It offers opportunities for the recognition of common human experience and individual feelings in a text; bibliotherapy has the potential to make people feel less alone. This recognition and potential improvement to wellbeing can be via diagnostic criteria and treatment suggestions, or via emotional insights.

Both models of bibliotherapy are currently mainly used with people with mild to moderate mental health issues, but there is increasing recognition that there is scope for it to be used more broadly with people with more enduring mental health conditions and with people with physical health conditions. The Reader's Shared Reading model is used in secure psychiatric hospitals to work with patients and the Reading Well scheme now includes collections of books for people with dementia and long-term health conditions (Farrington and Fearnley, 2010; The Reading Agency, 2015).

Why consider the role of narrative in bibliotherapy?

Storytelling is seen as a natural human act and an inescapable element of understanding lived experience (Frank, 2010). If stories are regarded as a ubiquitous phenomenon that helps to make life intelligible, then the question for bibliotherapy may be to consider how they can be used (Baker, 2004). Diverse fields of research, from English literature and medical sociology to psychology and neuroscience, are interested in how and why stories have such an effect on emotions and actions. Creating a narrative helps people to *make sense* of experience. Stories can help with meaning-making and improving understanding of human experience (Greenhalgh, 2016a). Some evidence suggests that it is the act of creating a narrative that is essential for increasing insight into actions and events (Pennebaker and Chung, 2011).

Thinking about the main features of a narrative can help to demonstrate why narratives and stories are important. Telling a story helps to shape experience by placing a structure on to it. This construction may be familiar: a story traditionally has a beginning, middle and an end. Learning from philosophy and history shows that the value of narratives is that they are time-bound (Ricoeur, 1974). This means that they have a plot, or are understood linearly (first this, then that, then another thing, then an end); as Carr (1986, 67) states: 'narrative is our primary (though not our only) way of organizing our experience of time.' Narratives also have a sense of ending, which provides the reader with some form of closure (Kermode, 1967).

People are more likely to remember stories than lists of events. This means that the impact of stories is likely to be more powerful than a statement of information (Greenhalgh, 2016a). However, narratives are not without artifice and imagination; telling a story about what happened to us is not necessarily to give a neutral account. A story is shaped by the person who is telling it, but it can also be affected by the person who is listening to or reading it. Placing the reader at the centre of understanding is important in bibliotherapy, and is one of the main elements of Reader Response Theory (Rosenblatt, 1938).

Illness narratives and autobiographies

When diagnosed with a health condition, people often try to seek information about this new diagnosis (Fallowfield and Ford, 1995; Litzkendorf et al., 2016). This information can be about causes, treatment and prognosis of the illness. However, it can be difficult to absorb and contain medical jargon. Often, medical information has a focus on managing symptoms, rather than containing information about what it is like to live day to day with a diagnosis or a condition. This knowledge of the day-to-day is often called *experiential knowledge* or *lived experience* and forms the basis of illness narratives. Illness narratives are usually written by patients who have experienced a mental or physical health condition (Bury, 2001). They are usually told about the impact of long-term physical and mental health conditions which may be life-changing, or even fatal, rather than more minor or acute (short-term) illnesses. These stories often draw on real-life experience rather being purely works of imagination.

In popular culture, there are many stories about health and illness, particularly within the genre of memoir and autobiography, where published accounts of health and illness are widely available. These accounts can be part of autobiographies which tell the story of someone's life in which illness may feature, or as *pathographies*, which tell the story of someone's illness (Kleinman, 1997).

According to the British Library's Public Lending Right loans of books by category for 2014/15 and 2015/16, biography and true story accounted for nearly 3% of library loans annually (the biggest categories being fiction (40%), children's (40%) and health and personal development (6%)) (British Library, 2016). It is not possible to break this figure down to look at how many titles would come into the sub-category of illness narratives – or to examine how many stories of illness are told within these wider life stories – but this does show the popularity of biography and life stories. Over recent years, several high-profile medical memoirs have also achieved significant acclaim – for example, Paul Kalanithi's book *When Breath Becomes Air* spent 12 weeks at the top of *The New York Times Non-Fiction Best Sellers* list in 2016. Reading people's stories of health and illness is a popular pastime.

Autobiographical accounts of illness sometimes describe the author's struggle with mental health problems, with famous titles including *An Unquiet Mind* by Kay Redfield Jamison, *Prozac Nation* by Elizabeth Wurtzel and William Styron's *Darkness Visible*. Annually, the Wellcome Collection in London awards the Wellcome Book Prize, which aims to showcase books that engage with aspects of health and medicine either in fiction or non-fiction. Several of these titles have been written by patients sharing their stories and other titles, including the 2016 prize winner Suzanne O'Sullivan's *It's All in Your Head*, share a clinician's perspective on patient experience.

Are illness narratives valuable for bibliotherapy?

While these titles may be popular, are these texts useful in bibliotherapy? If bibliotherapy aims to provide a new perspective on a topic and to offer opportunities for the recognition of common human experience, illness narratives may fulfil this role. While medical management can help alleviate symptoms of an illness, often the day-to-day aspects of living are not taken into account and in practice, 'becoming an expert in coping with the disease is often painful and nasty' (Storni, 2015). These narratives often focus on the painful, human experience of illness, so reading about illness overcome – or otherwise – may encourage fear, rumination and even hypochondria. Alternatively, these narratives may help the reader to process difficult emotions and learn to cope with a health condition.

When people start to become patients, they may need to understand their health condition better to manage it. Management of symptoms is only one aspect; they may also need to learn to live with it. Some evidence suggests that patients use the autobiographical accounts of others to facilitate this living with. In Mazanderani, Locock and Powell (2013), patients discussed the distinction between the value of real-life stories and fictionalized accounts on the same topic. Autobiographies also performed a different function from the medical information that was given to patients. Perhaps, then, there is value in accounts of living with illness.

However, it should be noted that some illness narratives do not have what could be termed a traditional or expected 'happy ending'. While the aim of bibliotherapy is not necessarily to be uplifting – it can be about providing cathartic release rather than positive emotions – the trajectory of many illness narratives should be acknowledged when considering their use in bibliotherapy. Research has shown that when people are depressed, they may find it hard to read about experiences of depression (Brewster, 2011). It may also be true that someone with a diagnosis of cancer may not find reading books like John Diamond's *C: because cowards get cancer too*, or Paul Kalanithi's *When Breath becomes Air* (both of which end with the early death of the author) to be an uplifting, or even cathartic, experience. On the other hand, the reader may find some solace in the recognition of their own experience and in facing difficult situations.

Mapping and defining illness narratives

Arthur Frank was one of the first sociologists to theorize illness narratives (Frank, 1995). After experiencing cancer, Frank found that telling a story about his illness helped to make sense of experience and enabled the restoration of self-identity. Frank found himself lost in the field of medicine, in which people's stories were used as clinical material with the aim of diagnosis and treatment rather than being seen as a representation of experience. When a person undergoes treatment, they become a body, colonized by medicine and, for a time, their social context is lost. By exploring what it was be a person with cancer, rather than just accepting these changes to body, identity and biography, Frank found a way to understand and theorize his illness. His narrative also created a guide for others on similar pathways, which can be seen as making a contribution to a community of people experiencing illness (Frank, 1995). As part of this theoretical and sense-making work, Frank identified three types of narrative which formed a person's pathway through illness. These are known as the restitution, chaos, and quest narratives. Understanding these narratives may be useful for those interested in bibliotherapy as they map out the structures of experience as understood within the field of illness narratives. However, as Frank states:

> . . . in any illness, all three narrative types are told, alternatively and repeatedly. At one moment in an illness, one type may guide the story; as the illness progresses, the story becomes told through other narratives.
>
> (Frank, 2010, 76)

Thus, understanding the structure of illness narratives is complicated, as a person's story may not be neatly defined and straightforward. While the restitution, chaos and quest narratives can be identified within a story, the complexities of treatment, relapse and illness mean that the story does not just follow one narrative. People can get better, and worse, and better again.

While in a work of imaginative literature, the author may make an effort to give the story a defined beginning, middle and an end, these features of a story are often more difficult to identify in illness narratives.

Frank's three types of illness narrative

Understanding the three different types of illness narrative outlined may help those involved in bibliotherapy to identify the main message that the autobiographical story is communicating to the reader. First is the restitution narrative, in which a person moves from a state of health, through an illness, and back to their previous state of health. Within this type of narrative is an expectation from the person listening to or reading the story that, despite the unpleasantness of the illness, there will be a resolution – a form of happy ending. The restitution narrative is often seen as a story of hope in which medicine will triumph over disease and there is always something that can be done that takes a person one step closer to being restored to health. Restitution narratives imply that patients get better. This implied direction does not necessarily make allowances for ongoing health problems and occurrences that mean people do not recover.

Second is the chaos narrative, which runs counter to the restitution narrative by removing all sense of certainty and resolution. Chaos narratives can be seen as threatening as they imply a loss of control and purpose. In some ways, they are not narratives in the traditional sense, as when things are in chaos, they are not connected clearly and may instead seem to drift from one thing to the next. This kind of narrative may seem ominous or even frightening, but it may be familiar to people with multiple long-term conditions or complex neurological conditions such as dementia. Undergoing treatment (for example, chemotherapy) which has severe side effects may also facilitate a form of chaos narrative.

Third is the quest narrative, which Frank (1995) positions as the type of narrative most commonly told within published illness narratives. In a quest narrative, the person takes their illness experience and uses it, perhaps to find out how they face difficulties such as illness or to use their illness to call for social change. Quest narratives take the disruption of illness and turn it into something with a wider message. In this type of narrative, people are not changed by illness but instead have used illness to enable them to find out who they really were all along.

Further mappings of illness narratives

Alongside Frank's categorization of narratives, other scholars have also highlighted different forms of narrative structures. Some of these structures have elements in common with Frank's narratives: for example, the tragic or sad narrative has much in common with the chaos narrative; and the heroic or detective narrative resembles the quest narrative in which the challenge is overcome. Others, such as the comic, ironic, and satirical narratives seem to have less in common (Soundy et al., 2013). These narratives provide an alternative lens through which illness can be viewed and may also be useful framings for using autobiographical illness narratives in bibliotherapy. Narratives can also be structured according to their function (Bury, 2001). Narratives can be:

- contingent, or examining the causes and origins of a disease as well as the effects on daily life
- moral narratives, which focus on the changes in the person and their identity caused by illness
- core narratives, which explore the experience of illness and the meaning of suffering.

(Bury, 2001).

This categorization may be useful for bibliotherapy, in that identifying these functions may help to direct people to stories that might be useful for them at different times, depending what kind of information, guidance or clarification they are seeking.

Problems with illness narratives

Frank's (1995, 2010) categorization of illness narratives is useful for bibliotherapy, as it shapes understandings of the stories that can be told and how they are told. His exploration of the structure of narratives helps to demonstrate why people might want to read illness narratives, but it also problematizes them. In another example, the academic primary care physician Trish Greenhalgh explored her own illness narrative after being diagnosed with breast cancer and undergoing chemotherapy (Greenhalgh, 2016b). In looking for explanatory accounts, she found that the existing narratives on the topic 'overwhelmed and disappointed me'. Greenhalgh found that the stories that had previously been told were not reflective of her experiences of illness and treatment. When she could not find her own experiences represented within literature, she started to question why what had happened to her was so different from what others had experienced. For those facilitating bibliotherapy, trying to match reader to text may be problematic if the story has not been written.

In this instance, Greenhalgh was able to articulate these differences between existing narratives and her experience to tell her own story following her illness, but this option to publish an account is not always open. One problem with illness narratives is that they are only told by some authors or narrators. This means they can lack diversity. Illness narratives can be reductionist about the structural dimensions of life. For example, a family with a disabled child telling their story of the struggles they have faced may be more likely to be middle-class than in poverty. Discussions of financial hardship associated with illness may be absent and a family in poverty might find their experience to be very different (Blume, 2017). There is a danger in telling someone that they will find another person's story to be relevant and representative.

Working with illness narratives and people with illnesses can be complex because there may not be one coherent account of an event. This lack of coherence may be damaging. Illness narratives are sold on the expectation that telling a story might bring coherence to life; this might be difficult to reconcile with difficult experiences that do not resolve into a traditional narrative structure or a 'happy ever after'. Storytellers often have to come to terms with the story as a 'work in progress' and be able to accept that life continued despite an undesirable end to the narrative arc.

Telling some stories may not be helpful for patients: for example, the narrative of fighting an illness and having courage to overcome it (Kelly and Dickinson, 1997). While this narrative can be helpful for some patients, in that it encourages action in the face of adversity, for others it can be damaging. Using fighting as a metaphor in the context of terminal illness may be stigmatizing and lead to self-blame if the person is not able to fight. In this way, illness narratives are not helpful as a resource for bibliotherapy, as they encourage the use of metaphors. Talking about the body as a machine that is fixable or about a battle against a disease places the patient in a position of control that may not be an accurate reflection of a situation. Implicit in the idea that someone may be fighting a battle is that the battle can be won.

Telling stories or narratives can also be called form-finding (Strawson, 2004). Drawing on the idea that journalists and historians aim to provide an impartial account of events, form-finding acknowledges that this involves giving a structure to a description of what has happened. When we read newspapers, we are looking for the journalists to connect together the events and establish causality. While there is an obligation to stick to the recognized facts, there is also an acknowledgement that a degree of selection and processing of information will occur.

Illness narratives also present this kind of form-finding. The aim is to present an account, but this is always shaped by personal memory and perception of events. If analysing imaginative literature, we might talk about an 'unreliable narrator' but this is complicated in illness narratives as they intend to be an account that represents a person's lived experience (Strawson, 2004). Can we say they are unreliable? For the most part, the narratives discussed in this chapter are 'true' in that they are based on real life experiences. However, the line between fiction and memoir is blurred as authors sometimes frame their texts as fictionalized accounts of experience, such as Sylvia Plath's (1963) *The Bell Jar*. Similarly, James Frey's (2004) *A Million Little Pieces* was originally marketed as a memoir before it was shown to be a mostly fictional account of his life (Barton, 2006). When considering their use in bibliotherapy, care needs to be taken to present these stories to readers appropriately.

Narrative medicine

Alongside illness narratives, many clinicians are also interested in storytelling within the field of narrative medicine. Some clinicians came to the conclusion that the use of evidence from clinical trials in medicine was leading to explanatory models of health and illness that ignored the individual experience of the patient. Medical professionals primarily took a biomedical, symptom-based model of health and illness and patients were seen as problems to be solved or machines to be fixed. Looking back over the history of medicine shows how relationships between doctors, patients and treatment has changed and developed. Before the 20th century, there were very few interventions that medical professionals could offer that would make a significant difference to the lives of patients. At this time, the rapport between doctor and patient was prized and relationships were the key to medicine: the traditional view of a bedside manner. As medicine changed and progressed, with the rise of laboratory medicine, germ theory and treatments like antibiotics and laparoscopic surgery, clinicians were able to make meaningful interventions to extend the life of their patients. As treating the symptoms became possible, the role of the doctor–patient relationship lessened (Bynum, 2008).

Modern medicine is more evidence-based, scientific and robust than ever before. However, this has led some clinicians to be concerned that medicine is no longer placing the patient at the heart of what is being done. Moving away from an evidence-based construction of medicine and towards a narrative-based one may help clinicians to remember to be patient-centred (Bury, 2001). Narrative medicine aims to help clinicians to understand patients in their own context. It encourages considering a more holistic view of health. The movement for narrative medicine is an international one and focuses on the cultural contexts of health, with a recognition that to ignore the history and social context of a patient means that the clinician may miss something important in their diagnosis (Greenhalgh, 1999).

Rita Charon, an American physician who was influential in the development of narrative medicine, highlighted that listening to patients' stories of illness and caregivers' narratives helped her to better understand her patients (Charon, 2006). As medicine became more technical and procedural, she was concerned that it was also becoming more impersonal. Her experience was that biological knowledge was being prioritized over empathy and respect for patients. Narrative medicine takes the view that this construction of knowledge about patients based purely on their symptoms is not enough to be able to successfully treat them. Instead, it draws on other academic disciplines; both work on illness narratives in sociology, and the role of fiction and poetry in the humanities make a contribution to medical knowledge.

In her text *Narrative Medicine* Charon (2006) paints a picture of the role of the stories told by both patients and clinicians. Both are interested in finding a cure for a disease, and while the clinician often focused on diagnosis, the patient also sought meaning – they wanted to understand how and why they were ill. This can be characterized as the 'voice of medicine' against the 'voice of the lifeworld' (Hurwitz and Charon, 2013). Listening to stories helped to create a more effective and compassionate medicine, in which the human response to illness was recognized. Understanding the patient perspective on illness was also recognized as having the potential to improve adherence to treatment. In defining the concept of narrative competence, the role of the clinician was changed (Charon, 2006). Good clinicians did not just treat the patient, but also understood what patients were going through and helped to illuminate that experience.

Narrative medicine thus became a matter of good ethical practice; if one did not listen to a patient then one could not fully diagnose and try to cure. Listening to patient stories can help to remind clinicians of the underpinning principles of medical practice (Hurwitz, 2015). For example, the principle of beneficence, or undertaking actions that aim to do good rather than to do harm to a patient, is supported by understanding their perspective and experiences (Hurwitz, 2015). Narrative medicine, with its focus on the relationship between finding out what someone's illness is and understanding how it fits with their life, can be associated with more compassionate care (Greenhalgh and Hurwitz, 1999). Following recent healthcare scandals in the UK, such as the poor care at the heart of the Mid-Staffordshire scandal, unnecessary deaths at Morecambe Bay and the abuse at Winterbourne View, the call for compassion in medicine is still present (Crowther et al., 2013; Francis, 2013).

This may be where hospital librarians can play a role in helping clinicians to engage with the principles of good-quality compassionate care. Hospital libraries are responsible for helping clinical staff keep up to date with medical developments and communicating information. This could extend to encouraging clinical staff to engage with narrative medicine or illness narratives to remind them of the value of compassion in healthcare. However, it is vital to remember that while reading has the potential to change attitudes for the better, this outcome is not guaranteed (Ahlzen, 2010).

Since 2015, the medical journal *The Lancet* has had a column examining the value that literature can bring to medicine (Marchalik and Jurecic, 2015). Drawing on imaginative literature (fiction) as well as illness narratives by authors including Paul Kalanithi and Oliver Sacks, the *From Literature to Medicine* format aims to demonstrate what can be learned from going beyond diagnoses and into narratives. Nevertheless, healthcare does not find narratives easy to deal with (Charon, 2006; Greenhalgh, 1999). Medicine likes to deal with definites and diagnosis, so positioning the diverse, contradictory stories of patients within this field is difficult.

Bringing together bibliotherapy, illness narratives and narrative medicine

From the overview of the literature presented here, we can start to see that there may be important connections between bibliotherapy, illness narratives and narrative medicine. Telling stories about health and illness might have a positive benefit for people telling stories and people hearing them. However, as this chapter has shown, this is not an uncomplicated process.

Because all narrativization is in some way a construction (we 'tell' a story), it may not be helpful to separate out fictional and autobiographical accounts. While there is some evidence that understanding lived experience as accessed via autobiography is helpful for understanding a condition (for example, see Mazanderani, Locock and Powell, 2013), there is also strong evidence that reading fictional narratives has a positive effect on increasing our understanding.

However, bibliotherapy aims to support people to reach a position of self-understanding, and the stories that people tell about their health and illness based on their experience might provide one route to better understanding. Illness narratives can enable people to understand their own illness more clearly, and they can also allow clinicians to understand illnesses better. They may also be useful for the friends and family of the person experiencing illness, helping them to better understand a condition. This may be particularly true in an illness like dementia, where carers have written accounts of their lives with someone experiencing severe symptoms and the emotional impact of this condition on their life.

Telling a story can be empowering for the person who tells it. It gives voice to someone's experience, and this can be very important in the face of difficult experiences. It can enable people to make sense of what has happened to them.

The existence of illness narratives may also encourage people to feel able to talk about their condition and not feel that they have to hide their symptoms. Some illnesses and medical conditions are still considered taboo or stigmatized and people do not feel able to talk about their experiences. Having a story told about a condition to some extent normalizes it and helps people to see that they are not the only person to feel a certain way or experience a particular situation. Such stories have been identified as helpful for people with mental health conditions (Brewster, 2011).

Sometimes, people find information in imaginative literature and fiction books (Sheldrick Ross, 1999). The value of reading narratives and identifying familiar situations or emotions in literature is a key concept for bibliotherapy (Gray et al., 2015). Information-seeking is not just searching for information and having a defined 'problem situation'; instead, information-seeking can be a more everyday process, with the 'incidental acquisition' of information (Sheldrick Ross, 1999). When people are coping with a long-term condition or difficult diagnosis, they may find this information encountering to be more conducive to locating relevant information to help support them than by going to look for clinical and factual information (Erdelez, 1999). Finding information about how others have represented a familiar experience or emotion, or coped with a similar situation, may be what is required, and it may be here that illness narratives and bibliotherapy connect.

For public librarians, what can be learned from illness narratives is that there might be a role for them to connect people with stories that can help to navigate the difficulties of illness. Some of this work has started to be done in the Reading Well Books on Prescription scheme, where memoirs of illness are used as tools to explain the experience of some long-term conditions. For medical and hospital librarians, it is important to consider the value of illness narratives and narrative medicine for clinicians, and to consider providing explanatory accounts of illnesses that people can use to increase their understanding of medical conditions. With recent calls to have a more compassionate stance towards care, it might be that illness narratives have a role to play.

Illness narratives may help us to see that when someone is diagnosed with a condition, their information needs may be diverse and not just related to symptom management. Thinking about helping people to meet their emotional needs in the face of illness may demonstrate how these stories may play a role in bibliotherapy.

References

Ahlzen, R. (2010) *Why Should Physicians Read? Understanding clinical judgement and its relation to literary experience*, Durham University, http://etheses.dur.ac.uk/343/%0D.

Baker, L. M. (2004) Information Needs at the End of Life: a content analysis of one person's story, *Journal of the Medical Library Association: JMLA*, **92** (1), 78–82.

Barton, L. (2006) The Man who Rewrote his Life, *The Guardian* (15 September), www.theguardian.com/books/2006/sep/15/usa.world.

Billington, J., Dowrick, C., Robinson, J., Hamer, A. and Williams, C. (2010) An Investigation into the Therapeutic Benefits in Relation to Depression and Wellbeing, University of Liverpool and Liverpool Primary Care Trust, www.thereader.org.uk/investigation-therapeutic-benefits-reading-relation-depression-well

Blume, S. (2017) In Search of Experiential Knowledge, *Innovation: the European journal of social science research*, **30** (1), 91–103.

Brewster, L. (2009) Books on Prescription: bibliotherapy in the United Kingdom, *Journal of Hospital Librarianship*, **9** (4), 399–407.

Brewster, L. (2011) (Brewster, E. A.) *An Investigation of Experiences of Reading for Mental Health and Wellbeing and their Relation to Models of Bibliotherapy*, PhD thesis, University of Sheffield, http://etheses.whiterose.ac.uk/2006.

Brewster, L. (2016) More Benefit from a Well-stocked Library than a Well-stocked Pharmacy: how do readers use books as therapy? In Rothbauer, P. M., Skjerdingstad, K. I., McKechnie, L. E. F. and Oterholm, K. (eds), *Plotting the Reading Experience: theory/policy/politics*, Wilfred Laurier University Press.

British Library (2016) *Public Lending Right: loans of books by category (%s) 2014/15–2015–16*, www.plr.uk.com/mediaCentre/loansByCategory/2015–2016ByCategory.pdf.

Bury, M. (2001) Illness Narratives: fact or fiction?, *Sociology of Health and Illness*, **23** (3), 263–85.

Bynum, W. F. (2008) *The History of Medicine: a very short introduction*, Oxford University Press.

Carr, D. (1986) *Time, Narrative, and History*, Indiana University Press.

Chamberlain, D., Heaps, D. and Robert, I. (2008) Bibliotherapy and Information Prescriptions: a summary of the published evidence-base and recommendations from past and ongoing Books on Prescription projects, *Journal of Psychiatric and Mental Health Nursing*, **15** (1), 24–36.

Charon, R. (2006) *Narrative Medicine: honoring the stories of illness*, Oxford University Press.

Crowther, J., Wilson, K. C. M., Horton, S. and Lloyd-Williams, M. (2013) Compassion in Healthcare – lessons from a qualitative study of the end of life care of people with dementia, *Journal of the Royal Society of Medicine*, **106** (12), 492–7.

Dowrick, C., Billington, J., Robinson, J., Hamer, A. and Williams, C. (2012) Get into Reading as an Intervention for Common Mental Health Problems: exploring catalysts for change. *Medical Humanities* **38** (1), 15–20.

Erdelez, S. (1999) Information Encountering: it's more than just bumping into information, *Bulletin of the American Society for Information Science*, **25** (3), 26–9.

Fallowfield, L. and Ford, S. L. (1995) No News is Good News: information preferences of patients with cancer, *Psycho-oncology*, **4** (3), 197–202.

Farrington, G. and Fearnley, D. (2010) Experiments in Reading: finding the middle ground between literature and psychiatry, *Madness and Literature: 1st international health humanities conference*, 6–8 August, Nottingham.

Francis, R. (2013) *Report of the Mid Staffordshire NHS Foundation Trust Public Inquiry*, www.gov.uk/government/publications/report-of-the-mid-staffordshire-nhs-foundation-trust-public-inquiry.

Frank, A. W. (1995) *The Wounded Storyteller: body, illness, and ethics*, University of Chicago Press.

Frank, A. W. (2010) *Letting Stories Breathe: a socio-narratology*, Chicago University Press.

Frey, J. (2004) *A Million Little Pieces*, John Murray.

Gray, E., Kiemle, G., Davis, P. and Billington, J. (2015) Making Sense of Mental Health Difficulties through Live Reading: an interpretative phenomenological analysis of the experience of being in a reader group, *Arts & Health*, **3015** (May), 1–14.

Greenhalgh, T. (1999) Narrative Based Medicine: narrative based medicine in an evidence based world, *British Medical Journal*, **318** (7179), 323–5.

Greenhalgh, T. (2016a) *Cultural Contexts of Health: the use of narrative research in the health sector*, Health Evidence Network Synthesis report 49, www.euro.who.int/__data/assets/pdf_file/0004/317623/HEN-synthesis-report-49.pdf?ua=1.

Greenhalgh, T. (2016b) Adjuvant Chemotherapy: an autoethnography, *Subjectivity*, **10** (4), 340–57.

Greenhalgh, T. and Hurwitz, B. (1999) Narrative Based Medicine: why study narrative?, *British Medical Journal*, **318** (7175), 48–50.

Hurwitz, B. (2015) Medical Humanities and Medical Alterity in Fiction and in Life, *Journal of Medical Ethics*, **41** (1), 64–7.

Hurwitz, B. and Charon, R. (2013) A Narrative Future for Health Care, *The Lancet*, **381** (9881), 1886–7.

Kelly, M. P. and Dickinson, H. (1997) The Narrative Self in Autobiographical Accounts of Illness, *The Sociological Review*, **45** (2), 254–78.

Kermode, F. (1967) *The Sense of an Ending: studies in the theory of fiction*, Oxford University Press.

Kleinman, A. (1997) *Writing at the Margin: discourse between anthropology and medicine*, University of California Press.

Litzkendorf, S., Babac, A., Rosenfeldt, D., Schauer, F., Hartz, T., Luhrs, V., Schulenburg, J. M. and Frank, M. (2016) Information Needs of People with Rare Diseases – what information do patients and their relatives require?, *Journal of Rare Disorders*, **2** (2), 1–11.

Marchalik, D. and Jurecic, A. (2015) Novel Remedies. *The Lancet*, **386** (10000), 1223.

Mazanderani, F., Locock, L. and Powell, J. (2013) Biographical Value: towards a conceptualization of the commodification of illness narratives in contemporary healthcare, *Sociology of Health and Illness*, **35** (6), 891–905.

Pennebaker, J. W. and Chung, C. K. (2011) Expressive Writing and its Links to Mental and Physical Health, *The Oxford Handbook of Health Psychology* 78712. 417–37.

Plath, S. (1963) *The Bell Jar*, Faber and Faber.

Ricoeur, P. (1974) Metaphor and the Main Problem of Hermaneutics, *New Literary History*, **6** (1) 95–110.

Rosenblatt, L. M. (1938) *Literature as Exploration*, Heinemann.

Sheldrick Ross, C. (1999) Finding without Seeking: the information encounter in the context of reading for pleasure, *Information Processing and Management*, **35** (6), 783–99.

Soundy, A., Smith, B., Dawes, H., Pall, H., Gimbrere, K. and Ramsay, J. (2013) Patient's Expression of Hope and Illness Narratives in Three Neurological Conditions: a meta-ethnography, *Health Psychology Review*, **7** (2), 177–201.

Storni, C. (2015) Patients' Lay Expertise in Chronic Self-care: a case study in type 1 diabetes, *Health Expectations*, **18** (5), 1439–50.

Strawson, G. (2004) Against Narrativity, *Ratio*, **16,** 428–52.

The Reading Agency (2015) *Reading Well: Books on Prescription*, http://reading-well. org.uk.

4

Bibliotherapy and graphic medicine

Sarah McNicol

Introduction

While most bibliotherapy activities focus on the use of written text, whether in the form of novels, poetry or self-help books, in recent years there has been a growing interest in the use of graphic novels and comics as a mode of bibliotherapy. The term 'graphic narratives' is used in this chapter to include both graphic novels and shorter comics in both print and digital formats. The chapter explores the ways in which graphic narratives of various types might be used as an effective form of bibliotherapy. It considers how the medium can be particularly effective in supporting important features of bibliotherapy such as providing reassurance, connection with others, alternative perspectives and models of identity. It then draws on examples of bibliotherapy collections from different library settings to demonstrate some of the ways in which graphic narratives are currently used in bibliotherapy practice, or might have potential to be used in the future. Finally, it considers the possible challenges of using graphic narratives for bibliotherapy, and how these could be overcome.

The representation of medical practices and conditions in graphic narratives is not new. For example, North American comic books of the 1940s were used to illustrate the history of medicine for mass audiences. Public health educators have used graphic narratives to communicate information on health issues for many years, including mental health (New York State Department of Mental Hygiene, 1950), the dangers of smoking (American Cancer Society, 1965), skin cancer (Putnam and Yanagisako, 1982) and HIV/AIDS (Gillies, Stork and Bretman, 1990). The number of graphic narratives being published on health-related issues appears to be growing however (Czerwiec et al., 2015). The last 15–20 years have seen the publication of a number sophisticated graphic narratives exploring health-related issues.

Many have experienced high levels of popularity among mainstream audiences, as well as critical acclaim. Examples include, David B's *Epileptic* (2005); Brian Fies' *Mom's Cancer* (2006); and Nicola Streeten's *Billy, Me and You: a memoir of grief and recovery* (2011), to name but a few. These texts are typically autobiographical, or semi-autobiographical, works created by skilled comics artists who have had a personal experience with illness, or with caring for a relative with a health condition. These types of texts are very different from what many people traditionally think of as 'comics'. Far from being light-hearted stories for children, these works are aimed at an adult audience and, whilst they often make use of humour, they explore serious and complex issues. As the potential of graphic narratives to address health-related issues becomes more widely recognized, the term that is increasingly being used to describe this activity is 'graphic medicine' (Williams, 2012). Over the last decade, a graphic medicine community has become established to explore the use of graphic narratives within healthcare; this includes clinicians and other healthcare professionals, artists and writers, publishers, librarians, researchers and others.

Reading graphic narratives

The majority of graphic medicine texts are, therefore, not simply easy-reading materials aimed at children or people with less developed literacy skills; they are, in fact, highly complex compositions that require well developed literacy. Graphic narratives can place a great demand on cognitive skills, as readers are required to interpret not only text, but also images (Chute, 2008). Comics differ from illustrated books in that the images are an essential element; they are not supplementary as in an illustrated text, but play an integral role in the telling of the story. This use of both text and image offers a 'combination of linguistic and visual codes' (Groensteen, 2007, 3), which is commonly described as creating 'more than the sum of its parts'.

The reader of a graphic narrative has been described as the author's 'silent accomplice' and 'equal partner in crime' (McCloud, 1994, 68). This links closely with Louise Rosenblatt's transactional theory of reading, in which a literary work is conceived not as an object, but as an experience shaped by the reader under the guidance of the text (and its author). Rosenblatt (1994, 25) proposes that a 'literary work exists in a live circuit set up between reader and text'. In reading a graphic narrative, however, the situation is more complex, as there are three components: reader, written text and images. Each person not only has their own reaction to a word based on personal experience and background, but also their own individual reaction to each icon in a picture. The reader creates an overall meaning by relating both the words and images to their own experiences. The result is that there is no single 'correct' or absolute meaning, but a series of more or less equally valid alternative interpretations. Furthermore, meaning is not fixed; it can change during the course of reading and can be modified after the work has been read. An important feature of graphic narratives, therefore, is the way in which they 'seem to allow more leeway in terms of meaning' (Williams, 2012, 25). They do not present a single, indisputable message, but instead rely on the reader to produce their own interpretation of the text and images. Of course, the author can guide the reader or offer 'clues'. An example is encouraging the reader to view an image in a certain way according to features of the layout, such as looking up at something to make it appear oppressive or frightening. However, even when such suggestions are offered, the reader still has some latitude in the way in which they construct meaning from the image. This freedom to interpret graphic narratives in a variety of ways, arguably, makes them ideally suited to certain types of bibliotherapy, particularly models that emphasize the importance of group discussion.

When reading a graphic narrative, it is important to remember that text and pictures do not necessarily convey the same message. For example, the picture might show a character's outward behaviour, while a thought bubble conveys their true feelings. Furthermore, even if image and text appear to be telling the same story, they do not necessarily present events at the same time, in the same order or from the same viewpoint. The process of deciphering the multiple messages that may be conveyed is, therefore, less straightforward than it might first appear. Pictures are often described as a type of 'received information' in contrast to words which have meanings that need to be 'perceived' (McCloud, 1994, 49). Thus, pictures are taken to be open and easily understood, whilst words are more abstract. Yet in graphic narratives, the worlds of words and pictures are brought together. As McCloud (1994, 49) argues, when words become bolder and more direct, they are 'received faster, more like pictures'. Likewise, pictures can appear as abstract and symbolic as words. For example, caricature, which is a common feature of comics, is said to be able to communicate more powerfully than 'the real thing' (Medley, 2010, 54). By removing realistic detail, other aspects of characters can be emphasized or imposed, which in turn, highlight connections or relationships that are less apparent in more literal or realistic images. Icons are another way in which pictures become more abstract or symbolic. These include universal icons, such as a circle with two dots and a line to represent a face, as well as culturally based conventions, such as dollar signs to represent money (Bamford, 2003). To read graphic narratives, readers have to understand both types of icons as well as comics-specific conventions, for example, streaking effects to indicate motion and balloons to indicate speech. Regular readers of comics naturally become more skilled in interpretation of such icons with practice.

All these features mean that the way in which information is coded in graphic narratives can be highly complex. Readers are required to interpret not only text, but also images and must, therefore, negotiate two systems of codes, or 'dual narrative tracks' (Chute, 2008, 452), which sometimes function independently and at other times interact. As a hybrid word-image format, graphic narratives require the reader to develop a number of strategies to make sense of the various possibilities presented. However, this also means that graphic narratives can offer the reader many options to form their own interpretation and make connections between the text and their own experiences. This can have powerful potential within bibliotherapy contexts, as discussed below.

Reading graphic medicine narratives

Considering the reading of graphic medicine narratives specifically, the fact that comics readers are encouraged to construct their own meaning means it is often easy for patients, or those close to them, to find resonances between the characters portrayed and their own lives when reading a narrative about a condition they suffer from. From here, it is almost inevitable that the act of reading a text will have practical implications. For instance, it can lead the reader to not only question their own feelings and reactions, but also the implications of these for the ways in which they act and react to others. Graphic narratives have been argued to be 'a very non-threatening medium' as well as a 'personalising medium' (McAllister, 1992, 18), one which 'universalises the illness experience' (Green and Myers, 2010). The fact that graphic narratives can effectively portray both actions and feelings means they 'may be a very effective tool in creating empathy and compassion' (Green and Myers 2010).

Williams (n.d.) argues that graphic narratives can be used as a resource for health professionals, as they play a valuable role in: reflecting or changing cultural perceptions of medicine; relating the subjective patient/carer/provider experience; enabling discussion of difficult subjects; and helping other sufferers or carers. Within healthcare consultations, graphic narratives might be used to initiate a discussion about a topic that is difficult to address verbally; they can allow patients' voices to be heard in alternative, and potentially powerful, ways; and they may empower patients to take greater control over their interactions with healthcare professionals. By showing different viewpoints in an accessible way, graphic narratives can encourage the reader to reassess their own attitudes and assumptions. This can be empowering for patients and illuminating for family members and wider society. In this way, these types of texts have the potential to challenge the stigma associated with many types of illness.

In a recent study of readers of health information comics (McNicol, 2017), interviewees were able to empathize with characters in the stories and some felt that this personal link helped them to relate to, and respond to, the information better than might have been the case had it been presented in a more impersonal way. Related to this idea of empathy was the notion that graphic narratives can provide a sense of companionship, reassurance and recognition through the realization that others were dealing with the same issues. Interviewees also thought that the visual metaphors and analogies presented could be helpful in explaining complex ideas in an easily understandable and memorable way. The graphic narratives studied could also lead to increased self-awareness; help to raise awareness of a condition; or be used to open up a discussion with healthcare professionals or family members. Interviewees reported that key features, such as the use of images, characterization and narrative, not only make complex issues easier to understand, but they also enable the reader to relate more closely to the conditions being discussed, allowing them to either gain greater self-awareness of their own situation or be able to better empathize with family members. As demonstrated in Chapter 2, typical reader reactions to graphic narratives display each of the three stages of bibliotherapy: identification, catharsis and insight. In fact, it might be argued that the abstract, or caricatured, nature of graphic narratives means it is easier for the reader to put themselves in the position of the character and relate their experiences to their own life than might be possible with more realistic representations. As McCloud (1994, 36) explains, ' . . . when you look at a photo or realistic drawing of a face—you see it as the face of another. But when you enter the world of the cartoon—you see yourself'.

Having explored the experience of reading graphic narratives, and graphic medicine texts in particular, the following section looks at the current availability of such texts in libraries.

Graphic narratives in libraries

In recent years, graphic narratives have become a common part of library collections and can have a high impact on circulation figures. In fact, Schneider (2014, 68) describes graphic novels as 'a near-ubiquitous part of public libraries today'. In surveys in the USA, around 98% of public libraries reported having graphic narratives in their collection (Schneider, 2014). Even in university libraries, there is considerable interest in graphic novels; Gavigan (2014, 99) reports a librarian from Columbia University who claims graphic novels are the most frequently requested material in the library's Ivy League request system. This has not always been the case, however; in the past, there has been notable opposition to the provision of graphic narratives in libraries. Throughout their history, graphic narratives have been viewed as 'the lowest rung of the cultural ladder' (Weiner, 2003, 3). Being on the margins, rather than in the mainstream of culture, they have long been viewed as objectionable or dangerous. Graphic narratives are still the subject of controversy today. For example, the graphic novels, *This One Summer* (Tamaki and Tamaki, 2014) and *Drama* (Telgemeier, 2012) were the two most frequently challenged books of 2016 according to the American Library Association's Office of Intellectual Freedom (American Library Association, 2017). It is worth noting that a number of the controversies surrounding graphic narratives have resulted from particular books being promoted among age groups for which they were not originally intended, for example by shelving adult graphic narratives in the children's section of libraries or bookshops. This points to a more pervasive problem, namely, a limited understanding and knowledge of graphic narratives among some librarians who are not regular readers of the medium. In the case of graphic medicine in particular, it is important to stress that, while there are titles aimed at children (for example the Medikidz[1] series), many of the texts are clearly targeted towards an adult audience.

Graphic medicine in libraries

Whilst general collections of graphic narratives are now common in libraries, specialized graphic medicine collections are much less frequently found. In a study to identify graphic medicine resources across the Greater Midwest Region in the USA, Noe (2015) only discovered a single graphic medicine collection: Ypsilanti District Library's collection includes around 90 titles covering a wide range of conditions and seven book club kits. Searching for three of the core titles in the field in university libraries

(*Epileptic* (David B, 2005), *Mom's Cancer* (Fies, 2006) and *Graphic Medicine Manifesto* (Czerwiec et al., 2015)), Noe found that only two of the eleven libraries searched had all three titles and two had none of them in their collections.

Examples of graphic medicine collections can be found, however. The Bibliothèque de la Santé (Health Library) at the Université de Montréal in Canada started to develop a graphic medicine/graphic science collection in 2011 and by 2017 had a collection of over 100 titles (Clar and Brault, 2013). This collection has been integrated into a number of courses within the university. For example, titles have been added to course outlines; introduced with preparatory activities for courses; and included within e-learning modules. In 2017, the library started an outreach collection in the Faculty of Medicine students' lounge. Each month, the librarian selects ten comics from the Health Library collection which are then made available in the students' lounge for the current month. The hope is that this will allow more students to read the books and discover the potential of comics for developing a better understanding of patients and their families, as well as providing educational material for patients.

The Newcomb Library in the UK is a small National Health Service (NHS) library serving staff and students at Homerton University Hospital in London. It has growing collection of over 30 graphic novels, many of which were donated by a former consultant. This 'Get Graphic' collection is described as 'a unique resource within NHS libraries' (Newcomb Library, 2016). It forms part of the library's efforts to provide a broader range of materials than might be expected in a hospital library: for example, novels with a medical theme and health-related board games. Many of the graphic medicine titles focus on mental health issues, but other topics such as cancer and bereavement are also covered. When the collection was initially established, a small exhibition was held in the library to raise awareness and the titles were added to the library catalogue. Rather than having a separate graphic novels collection, the library classifies and shelves the books with others on the same topic. While some library users who have borrowed from the collection read the graphic medicine titles for their own enjoyment or relaxation, others have used them with patients. The library is continuing to gradually build the collection and hopes to organize a graphic medicine event bringing together authors and clinicians in the future.

One of the most developed graphic medicine resources is that at the Lamar Soutter Library at the University of Massachusetts Medical School in the USA. Although this library only began to develop a graphic medicine collection in

2016, it now has around 70 graphic narratives, as well as a number of Graphic Medicine Book Kits that include six copies of a graphic novel; a quick guide to reading graphic narratives; discussion questions; and topic-relevant MedlinePlus information (Noe, 2017). As not everyone who requests a kit has run a book club before, the librarian responsible for the development of the kits provides support with the process of running an effective book club. There are currently eleven book club kits available for loan by any organization in New England on ten topics: addiction (two kits), aging, AIDS, cancer, epilepsy, grief, LGBTQ, mental health, OCD, and veterans' health. As well as public and academic libraries, there have also been requests for kits from veterans' health organizations. As the project is relatively new, there is limited feedback from participants so far, but this type of resource clearly has considerable potential for bibliotherapy purposes. The library hopes to expand this service in the future: for example, developing kits focused on different forms of cancer or the needs of female, as well as male, veterans. As well as being loaned to reading groups, these book kits have been used within teaching in the university's medical school. In the short course, 'Health Literacy and Comics', students discuss the challenges of health literacy; gain an understanding of the basics of comics design; and examine the evidence for using graphic narratives in healthcare. They then use the book kits, and finally present a graphic narrative they have created themselves illustrating a clinical, or personal, experience of health. This exercise has resulted in some powerful narratives demonstrating how graphic medicine might help clinicians to better understand patients' experiences and perspectives.

Creating graphic narratives

The process of creating a graphic narrative, described above as part of the University of Massachusetts' course for medical students, could have wider application within bibliotherapy. As with prose and poetry, bibliotherapy can involve the creation of graphic narratives, as well as the consumption of those already published. For example, the 'Graphic Lives' project worked with a group of British-Bangladeshi women in Greater Manchester in the UK to support them in telling their life stories in the form of digital comics. The women took part in a series of activities[2] over approximately six months, culminating in the creation of finished comics. Most of the women had very limited English and it is unlikely they would have felt comfortable joining a traditional bibliotherapy group. However, through looking at examples of published comics and exploring different visual methods, they were able to explore complex, and sometimes traumatic, events in their lives. During the course of the project, it became evident that many of the women had experienced mental health issues such as anxiety or depression. While they found it hard to express the difficulties they had experienced in words (and particularly in English), the comics format gave them the freedom to explore other ways of communicating issues that affected their wellbeing. Incorporating images helped them to convey the emotions behind their experiences more effectively than words alone. For example, as shown in Figure 4.1, when one of the women, Fatima, wrote about her miscarriages, she did so in a quite matter-of-fact way. However, the page is filled with an image of a huge pram that pushes the text to the edge of the page and suggests how this experience overshadowed everything else in her life (Figure 4.1).

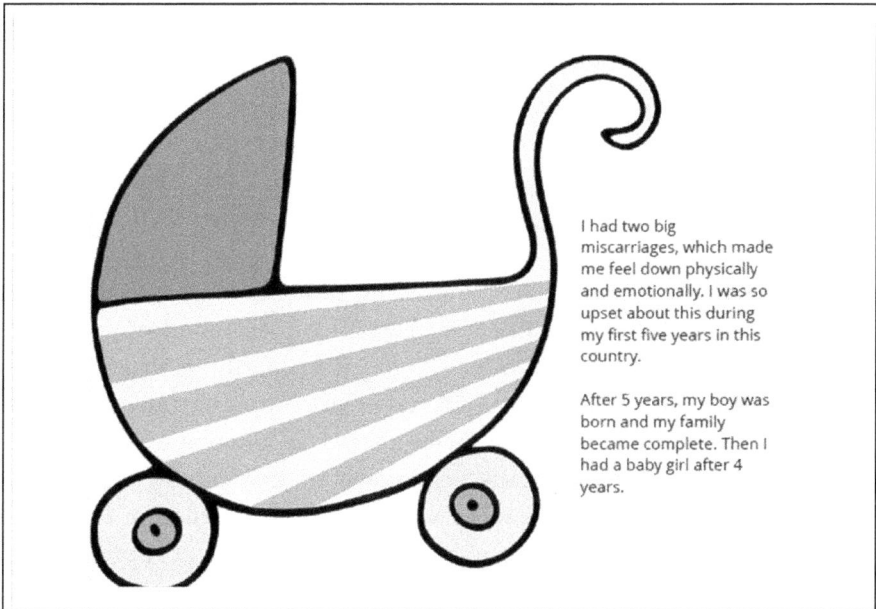

I had two big miscarriages, which made me feel down physically and emotionally. I was so upset about this during my first five years in this country.

After 5 years, my boy was born and my family became complete. Then I had a baby girl after 4 years.

Figure 4.1. *Page from Fatima's comic*

While this workshop was conducted for a research project, the process could be adapted for bibliotherapy groups, resulting in participants creating graphic narratives reflecting their experiences of living with (or caring for others with) a wide range of conditions, just as some groups, such as those described in Chapter 6 currently produce prose or poetry.

Challenges of using graphic narratives in bibliotherapy

This chapter has argued that graphic narratives have considerable potential within bibliotherapy. To date, however, they have been relatively underused: few libraries have graphic medicine collections and the possibilities for both reading groups and creative activities are only just starting to be explored.

Using graphic narratives as a form of bibliotherapy is not without its challenges, especially as many common bibliotherapy activities are designed to support the use of written texts. For example, graphic narratives can be difficult to use with read-aloud groups, as group members do not just need to hear the words, but also see the images. Sharing images may present practical difficulties, compounded by the fact that, while the facilitator can control the pace at which words are shared (taking account of the needs of the group), people are likely to want to 'read' images at their own speed.

A further barrier may be the fact that in many countries, including the UK and the USA, most adults do not regularly read graphic narratives and may not be comfortable with the medium. In the past, graphic medicine narratives have most commonly been seen as a technique to make information accessible for low-literacy patients (e.g. Toroyan and Reddy, 2005; Zielinski, 1986), young people or non-native speakers (Green and Myers, 2010). To some extent, this is still the case, despite the growing interest in more complex graphic narratives. This means that the full potential of graphic medicine within a wider population has not been fully explored. Many people's understanding of graphic narratives is based primarily on experiences of superhero and children's comics. The types of graphic narratives used for bibliotherapy purposes may not, therefore, match common expectations of the format and this could cause confusion or uncertainty. A common expectation is that graphic narratives will be light-hearted and trivial, so there may be a question for some as to whether the medium is appropriate to address serious health-related issues. It is possible that this may result in some initial resistance to the idea of using graphic narratives for bibliotherapy purposes. Furthermore, graphic narratives may not be as easy to read as they first appear. While some use straightforward traditional panel formats, others can have complex layouts that are more challenging for novice readers of the medium.

A further challenge is that bibliotherapy group facilitators may be less confident using graphic narratives. While they may be have a good knowledge of, and be proficient in using, written prose or poetry with bibliotherapy groups, facilitators may not have the same level of knowledge of graphic narratives and may also be unsure of the best ways to use these texts with groups.

Of course, as with written texts, caution needs to be exercised when selecting graphic narratives to use with bibliotherapy groups. When I shared a number of graphic narratives with a group of people with dementia, they felt that the design of some graphic narratives was ill-suited for people with dementia: for example, too much text on a page or a confusing layout. Moreover, reading the graphic narratives was quite a negative experience for this group, as they did not feel themselves to be adequately represented in the characters with dementia. Rather than the bleak picture painted in many texts, they wanted the overall message to be a more positive one that demonstrated that that living with the condition could have positive, as well as negative, aspects. This lack of identification with the characters limited the extent to which they were able to engage with the texts.

Identifying graphic narratives to add to library collections can be a challenge in itself. Whilst titles from mainstream publishers are easily available from bookshops or suppliers, other graphic medicine titles can be extremely difficult for librarians to source. Often, graphic narratives are not available through conventional library suppliers, but sold directly by creators either online or at comics fairs. While specialist booksellers such as 'Gosh!' and 'Page 45' do supply graphic narratives to school and public libraries, it obviously takes some knowledge of the field to identify suppliers such as these.

Finally, it is important to mention that digital comics are becoming increasingly common, especially within graphic medicine, where individuals who have experienced a health condition might set up a blog or web page to share comics about their experiences. Two well known examples of online comics are Allie Brosh's *Hyperbole and a Half*,[3] about the experience of depression, and Darryl Cunningham's *Psychiatric Tales*,[4] about his experiences working in mental health. Both these works started as blogs, although they were later published as printed books. There are many other lesser-known online graphic narratives about health conditions, but it can be extremely difficult for libraries to catalogue such resources and make them discoverable. Comics Plus[5] and similar resources allow libraries to offer users access to digital graphic narratives. However, searching Comics Plus reveals relatively few titles with a health focus. So, whilst digital comics hold future potential for bibliotherapy purposes, practical issues make them difficult to identify and use at present.

Conclusions

This chapter has argued that there is huge untapped potential for the use of graphic narratives for bibliotherapy. As Williams (2012, 25) describes, graphic medical narratives are usually consumed by readers with 'some sort of vested interest'. However, many health-focused graphic narratives have a much wider appeal, for example, Nicola Streeten's *Billy, Me and You* (2011) or Al Davidson's *The Spiral Cage* (2013), both of which made it onto a list of top graphic memoirs (Talbot and Talbot, 2012) alongside classics such as *Ethel and Ernest* (Briggs, 1998) and *Persepolis* (Satrapi, 2008). In addition, there are graphic novels that do not address health issues directly, but as in the case of prose novels, may be valuable texts for bibliotherapy purposes: for instance, Shaun Tan's (2007) wordless graphic narrative, *The Arrival*.

While theories of reading suggest that graphic narratives are highly suited to bibliotherapy activities, both attitudinal and practical barriers limit their use at present. Pilot projects, such as that at Lamar Soutter Library, give an indication of what might be possible, but work is needed to develop methods of bibliotherapy that can work for a graphic narrative format, and with diverse audiences. For bibliotherapy facilitators who feel less confident working with graphic narratives, one option may be to partner with someone with skills in visual literacy or comics – for example, a visual artist or a library colleague who runs a graphic novel reading club. Furthermore, the field is fortunate in having the vibrant and active Graphic Medicine[6] community, which can provide support and advice.

In summary, graphic medical narratives deserve wider consideration by those planning bibliotherapy interventions. Whilst the format may not be suitable for all individuals, or all situations, the potential benefits are considerable if the format is used appropriately. The first stage in developing greater use of graphic narratives in bibliotherapy is increased awareness amongst librarians, healthcare professionals and other bibliotherapy facilitators. My hope is that this chapter contributes to this wider recognition of the potential of graphic medicine among bibliotherapists.

Acknowledgements

Many thanks to Matthew Noe of Lamar Soutter Library at UMass Medical School for discussing his work to develop and support graphic medicine in the New England area and more widely. Thanks also to Kaye Bagshaw, Library Manager at Newcomb Library, Homerton University Hospital NHS Foundation Trust, for providing information about the development of the library's graphic medicine collection, and to Monique Clar, Bibliothécaire, Bibliothèque de la Santé, Université de Montréal for providing information on the latest developments in the library's graphic medicine collection.

Notes

1   www.jumohealth.com/products.
2   www.esriblog.info/wp-content/uploads/2017/08/About20the20project.pdf.
3   http://hyperboleandahalf.blogspot.co.uk.
4   http://darryl-cunningham.blogspot.co.uk.
5   https://library.comicsplusapp.com.
6   www.graphicmedicine.org.

References

American Cancer Society (1965) *Where There's Smoke*, Commercial Comics, Inc.
American Library Association (2017) *Top Ten Most Challenged Book Lists*, www.ala.org/advocacy/bbooks/frequentlychallengedbooks/top10#2016.
Bamford, A. (ed). (2003) The Visual Literacy White Paper, https://www.aperture.org/wp-content/uploads/2013/05/visual-literacy-wp.pdf
Briggs, R. (1998) *Ethel and Ernest: a true story*, Jonathan Cape.
Clar M. and Brault I. (2013) Graphic Medicine from Library to Classroom. Presented at CHLA/ABSC 2013: Inspiration Cooperation Innovation, 22–25 May, Saskatoon, Canada.
Chute, H. (2008) Comics as Literature? Reading graphic narrative, *Publication of the Modern Language Association of America (PMLA)*, **123** (2), 452–65.
Czerwiec, M. K., Williams, I., Squier, S. M., Green, M. J., Myers, K. R. and Smith S. T. (2015) *Graphic Medicine Manifesto*, Pennsylvania State University Press.
David B. (2005) *Epileptic*, Jonathan Cape.
Davidson, A. (2013) *The Spiral Cage*, Active Images.
Fies, B. (2006) *Mom's Cancer*, Abrams.
Gavigan, K. W. (2014) Shedding New Light on Graphic Novel Collections: a circulation and collection analysis study in six middle school libraries, *School Libraries Worldwide*, **20** (1), 97–115.
Gillies P. A., Stork A. and Bretman M. (1990), Streetwize UK: a controlled trial of an AIDS education comic, *Health Education Research*, **5** (1), 27–33
Green, M. J. and Myers, K. R. (2010) Graphic medicine: use of comics in medical education and patient care, *BMJ*, **340**, c863.
Groensteen, T. (2007) *The System of Comics*, University Press of Mississippi.

McAllister M. P. (1992) Comic books and AIDS, *Journal of Popular Culture*, **26** (2), 1–24.

McCloud S. (1994) *Understanding Comics: the invisible art*, Harper Collins.

McNicol, S. (2017), The potential of educational comics as a health information medium, *Health Information and Libraries Journal*, **34** (1), 20–31.

Medley, S. (2010) Discerning Pictures: how we look at and understand images in comics, *Studies in Comics*, **1** (1), 53–70.

New York State of Mental Hygiene (1950) *Blondie Comic Books*, New York Department of Mental Hygiene.

Newcomb Library (2016), *Learning is Serious Fun*, http://www.londonlinks.nhs.uk/events-2016/november/3-homerton-university-hospital-nhs-foundation-trust-please-fill-whole-page.pdf.

Noe, M. (2015) Graphic Medicine and Medical Libraries: a new opportunity. Presented at Greater Midwest Region, Medical Library Association Conference, Louisville, KY, http://works.bepress.com/matthewnoe/2.

Noe, M. (2017) Comics and Medicine: building collections and raising awareness, *Community Engagement and Research Symposia* **9**, http://escholarship.edu/chr_symposium/2017/posters/9.

Putnam, G. L., and Yanagisako, K. L. (1982) Skin Cancer Comic Book: evaluation of a public educational vehicle, *Cancer Detection and Prevention*, **5**, 349–56.

Rosenblatt, L. M. (1994) *The Reader, the Text, the Poem: the transactional theory of the literary work*, Southern Illinois University Press.

Satrapi, M. (2008) *Persepolis: the story of a childhood and the story of a return*, Vintage.

Schneider, E. F. (2014) A Survey of Graphic Novel Collection and Use in American Public Libraries, *Evidence Based Library and Information Practice*, **9** (3), 68–79.

Streeten, N. (2011) *Billy, Me and You: a memoir of grief and recovery*, Myriad Editions.

Talbot, B. and Talbot, M. (2012) Bryan and Mary Talbot's Top 10 Graphic Memoirs, *The Guardian*, 18 April, www.theguardian.com/books/2012/apr/18/bryan-mary-talbot-10-graphic-memoirs?CMP=twt_fd.

Tamaki, M. and Tamaki, J. (2014) *This One Summer*, First Second Books.

Tan, S. (2007) *The Arrival*, Hodder Children's Books.

Telgemeier, R. (2012) *Drama*, Graphix.

Toroyan, T. and Reddy, P. (2005) Participation of South African Youth in the Design and Development of AIDS Photo-comics, *International Quarterly of Community Health Education*, **25** (1), 149–63.

Weiner, S. (2003) *Faster than a Speeding Bullet: the rise of the graphic novel*, Nantier, Beal, Minoustchine.

Williams, I. C. M. (n.d.) *Why Graphic Medicine?*, Graphic Medicine, www.graphicmedicine.org/why-graphic-medicine.

Williams, I. C. M. (2012) Graphical Medicine: comics as medical narrative, *Medical Humanities*, **38** (1), 21–7.

Zielinski, C. (1986) Publishing for the Grass Roots—a comic book on immunization, *World Health Forum*, **7** (3), 273–7.

Part 2

Bibliotherapy case studies

5

Read to Connect: reading to combat loneliness and promote resilience

Natalia Tukhareli

Introduction

It has been more than a century since the term bibliotherapy was introduced to describe the practice of using literary materials to address mental health issues. Today, it is used as an umbrella term to cover a variety of clinical and non-clinical interventions involving books, reading and communication around texts. While psychologists share their positive experiences of using fiction and self-help materials in their counselling practices (Mendel, Harris and Carson, 2016; Volpe et al., 2015); librarians report on the success of collaborative Books on Prescription schemes in public libraries (Carty et al., 2016; Robertson et al., 2008); and facilitators of shared reading groups in community settings describe the psychological and social benefits of read-aloud sessions for diverse populations (Dowrick et al., 2012; Hodge, Robinson and Davis, 2007). Behind these academic reports and anecdotal stories are real people who were helped during difficult times in their lives.

My bibliotherapy journey went through different stages — from my personal experiences of the transformative power of literature, to an academic exploration of the art and science of bibliotherapy as a discipline, to first-hand observations of how books can improve the lives of individuals dealing with various life challenges, including those facing a terminal illness. Throughout my life, I have had many powerful moments of interaction with books, while recreating narrative worlds and building intellectual and emotional connections with their authors and characters. Books not only opened new perspectives and opportunities, but helped me to cope with difficult times in my life, including adjusting to the life in a new country while dealing with changes in career and family crisis. It was then when I came across a short story *The Road to Rankin's Point* by Alistair MacLeod, and this particular line: 'It does not matter that some things are difficult. No one has ever said that life is to be easy. Only that it is to be lived.' (MacLeod, 2000, 172). These words immediately resonated with another line from my favourite German poet Rainer Maria Rilke, who wrote in his *Letters to a Young Poet*: 'what matters is to live everything' (Rilke, 2011, 51). The therapeutic effect of these lines on me was so strong that it helped dismiss my fears and doubts and activate the inner resources for a new start in life.

A few years later, I used the same short story and the quote to address resilience and adversity when facilitating a reading group. These resources spoke to other individuals living through difficult times and triggered a meaningful discussion. What struck me back then was the fact that none of the group participants knew about these two authors. Moreover, they would have never come across these books if it had not been for our reading session. This episode turned into an important motivational moment for me and reinforced my enthusiasm for connecting books and people and expanding the value of reading to those who, for various reasons, did not have a chance to discover the joy of reading and experience its numerous benefits. Motivated by this goal and by the success of the bibliotherapy programme that I conducted at the Nkosi's Haven in Johannesburg, South Africa, I switched my focus from the theoretical exploration of literature to applying it to everyday life: from my academic research on concepts of loneliness and solitude in the poetry of Rainer Maria Rilke to connecting his writings with individuals who otherwise would never 'meet' the German poet whose deep insight into the nature of loneliness could guide those struggling with this human condition.

Jane Davis, the founding director of The Reader in the UK, shared a similar experience in her opinion piece 'Literature isn't a luxury but a life-changer' (Davis, 2017). In Davis' view the decision to 'get great books out of the university and into the hands of people who need them,' who would not otherwise come into contact with literature, motivated her to create The Reader and start 'a reading revolution.' Within a short period of time, her shared reading approach has expanded all over the UK and overseas and inspired many people, including myself, to get engaged in this form of creative bibliotherapy. This chapter focuses on several bibliotherapy programmes I have developed in South Africa and Canada, adapting the structure of a read-aloud programme to the needs of diverse populations, which has allowed me to introduce creative ways of using books and reading to promote wellbeing and resilience and combat social isolation.

Methodology: the exploration of theoretical and practical aspects of bibliotherapy

Underpinning the bibliotherapy projects described in this chapter is a methodology that includes an extensive literature review of the published bibliotherapy research and a case study of the Bibliotherapy Programme on HIV/AIDS that I developed and implemented in 2010 in Johannesburg, South Africa. The literature review covered a broad range of theoretical and practical aspects of bibliotherapy, from the academic discussion around the topics related to the transformative potential of literature, to the publications describing the bibliotherapy applications developed and implemented in various clinical and non-clinical settings in the UK and internationally (Tukhareli, 2014). This thorough analysis of the current theories and practices in bibliotherapy has provided the theoretical foundation and suggested practical steps to the development and the implementation of the reading programmes described in this chapter.

The literature review revealed an important quality of literary texts that defines their potential to encourage a therapeutic response from readers. Davis (2009) states that the premise of books' influence on people's minds and souls is that literature 'replicates more faithfully than any other man-made form the sense, structure, and feel of experience itself, while at the same time affording a safe distance from which to refract that experience.' This notion is supported by neuroscience research studies that show that imagining an act engages the same motor and sensory programmes in the brain that are involved in doing it (Doidge, 2007). Within this context, books can be viewed as an inexhaustible source of life experiences, which can be safely explored within the conventional boundaries of fiction. While exploring a broad range of life situations through the narratives of fictional stories, the reader has always a chance of 'living' their own situation through the narrative of the book. Therefore, as Cheu (2001, 39) asserts: 'the result of the bibliotherapeutic process is not a reading, but a writing and re-writing of the reader's own narrative – the recognition and the transformation of the reader's own voice through reading others' words.' This is where a positive change may occur. As Gold (2002, 126) notes, the wonderful thing about literature is that 'we do not have to be at physical or relational risk to gain increased knowledge of ourselves.'

The therapeutic potential of a creative book–reader interaction can be amplified when it takes place in a bibliotherapy group setting and becomes a 'collective action of the literature, facilitator, and group' (Dowrick et al., 2012, 19). By bringing together a diversity of independent viewpoints expressed in the text (Oatley, 1999) and voices of the individuals engaged into dynamic interactions with the text and with each other, a bibliotherapy group enhances the chance to 'find what you need in what you read' (Gold, 1990, 279). The academic literature highlights the benefits of shared reading groups run in diverse settings, including hospitals, mental health centres, neurological rehabilitation units, retirement homes, libraries, shelters and prisons. Although the reading programmes studied did not aim to achieve specific therapeutic goals, the evaluation reports describe improved mental, emotional, psychological and social wellbeing of shared reading group participants (Billington et al., 2014; Billington et al., 2010; Davis et al., 2012; Hodge, Robinson and Davis, 2007; Robinson, 2008a, 2008b; Robertson and Billington, 2013; Walsh, 2010). The findings of these studies are congruent with the outcomes of the bibliotherapy programme that I have facilitated at Nkosi's Haven, a recognized NGO offering holistic care and support for destitute HIV/AIDS-infected mothers, their children, and resulting AIDS orphans in Johannesburg, South Africa.

An HIV/AIDS bibliotherapy programme

During my three-month stay and volunteer work at Nkosi's Haven in the summer of 2010, I established a library for the residents of the shelter and conducted an innovative bibliotherapy programme on HIV/AIDS. The programme aimed to dispel the stigma associated with HIV/AIDS and assist in breaking the isolation and loneliness of the residents of the shelter. A total of 82 people (children and adults) participated in weekly read-aloud group sessions. While adopting the approach taken by creative bibliotherapy schemes in the UK (Get into Reading and RAYS in Kirklees Libraries), I integrated an educational component into the reading programme. Books used for bibliotherapy sessions included both fiction and non-fiction, such as short stories, prose excerpts, poetry, documented accounts of true stories told by people living with HIV/AIDS and educational resources on HIV/AIDS.

The case study described in earlier publications (Tukhareli, 2014; Tukhareli, 2011) investigated the educational and recreational benefits of bibliotherapy in relation to HIV/AIDS. The outcomes of the study showed that the bibliotherapy programme contributed to increased knowledge about HIV/AIDS and HIV-related issues; enhanced positive thinking and attitudes; reduced isolation and loneliness; and a reinforced sense of community. By the end of the programme, many children acknowledged an increase in their comfort level in thinking and talking about HIV/AIDS, while the adult participants (10 out of 23 women) developed action plans to make positive changes in their current situations. The participants' testimonies highlight the transformational effect that they experienced as a result of their involvement in reading sessions:

> It [the programme] has motivated me in so many ways – to love, to accept my status, to understand other mothers and to help one another.

> These sessions revealed something inside me. Now I know that everything is possible. As long as you don't give up.

The academic exploration of the science and art of bibliotherapy and my personal observations of the transformational effect of books on the residents of Nkosi's Haven have shaped my perspective on a bibliotherapy-based reading group as the space and place where fictional and non-fictional stories can be shared in a safe and caring environment to console, inspire, educate and guide through life crises and difficult transitions. In 2011, I launched the bibliotherapy project Read to Connect to address the challenges of everyday life through bibliotherapy and promote wellbeing, resilience and social inclusion to diverse populations of Toronto, Canada.

Reading for wellbeing and resilience: the bibliotherapy-based project in Toronto, Canada

This bibliotherapy-based reading project aimed to address existential, or 'living' problems, through thematic compilations of readings of various genres to promote individual and community health, wellbeing and resilience. The principal features of this approach include:

1 thematic compilations of literary materials to address existential themes (e.g. loneliness, adversity, forgiveness, happiness, love, resilience) and more specific topics relevant to the real-life situations that the programme participants may deal with in their lives (e.g. relocation, poverty, parenting, grief and bereavement, work-related stress)
2 reading materials of various genres, including both fiction and non-fiction: e.g. parables, short stories, novels, poetry, biographies, autobiographies, memoirs, letters, diaries, self-help books, academic manuscripts, research articles

3 the diversity of selected materials: readings from classical and contemporary authors representing different cultural and spiritual traditions
4 short reading pieces included compilations: short stories, poems, excerpts from novels and non-fiction books
5 the educational or informational component: these included non-fiction materials addressing healthy living tools, stress-management techniques and resilience-building strategies supported by the evidence-based research
6 delivery methods: *in-person* – shared reading groups in a library and community settings and *online* – the distribution of electronic copies of thematic compilations at workplace.

The approach was used in the Read to Connect and Bibliotherapy for Staff programmes developed and delivered in Toronto, Canada.

Read to Connect programme

The Read to Connect programme was developed for the clients of St John the Compassionate Mission, a non-profit organization supporting disadvantaged community members in Toronto. Delivered in 2011–2012, it involved reading and communication around texts in small groups. A total of 31 adults participated in the programme over a period of six months, with five people on average attending weekly reading sessions. The programme aimed to promote resilience, and break isolation and loneliness for people dealing with various life challenges such as unemployment and poverty; chronic medical conditions; life changes and adjustments (e.g. recent immigrants and refugees); loss and bereavement; family crisis; and parenting challenges.

The name Read to Connect reflected the view of bibliotherapy as an effective tool in helping individuals living through difficult times to reinforce or restore meaningful connections with themselves and with the world around. The specific themes – including loneliness and isolation, dealing with adversity, loss and grief, forgiveness, gratitude and appreciation, positive attitude, meaning in life, compassion, love and giving, self-acceptance, responsibility, family relationships, parenting and connection with nature – were identified and addressed through compilations of readings of various genres. As many participants could not commit to regularly attending the programme, our goal was to complete the readings and discussion on a specific topic in one session.

The innovative content of the Read to Connect programme was delivered within a shared reading model originally developed by The Reader. The reading session lasted for 1½ hours and included an introduction, reading aloud a selection of literary materials and a guided group discussion. Reading aloud is considered an important factor contributing to the accessibility of the programme to diverse populations groups, including individuals with low literacy skills and learning disabilities. During the initial implementation of the programme, one episode occurred that provides a good illustration of this. When inviting the clients of the St John the Compassionate Mission to join our weekly reading group, I received the following response from one person 'I don't want to read. I am not a good reader.' However, after I clarified that she did not have to read herself but only listen to me or other volunteers reading aloud, she joined the group and stayed until the end of the programme. The woman had a learning disability, but this did not prevent her from connecting to readings and participating in group discussions. Like many other participants of the programme, who were previously not engaged with books and reading, she could listen, reflect and share her thoughts and feelings triggered by the reading. This observation has supported the previously published evidence highlighting the benefits of the read-aloud component of shared reading groups (Hodge, Robinson and Davis, 2007; Davis 2009).

The reading materials were selected from a broad variety of both fiction and non-fiction texts, including parables, short stories, novels, poetry, biographies, autobiographies, memoirs, letters and manuscripts in the humanities and social sciences. Each compilation included on average five reading materials: a short story or an excerpt from a novel, one or two poems and two or three passages from non-fiction texts addressing the theme. By covering a few different readings during the session, the programme participants were given more opportunities to connect to readings and get involved into discussion. Prior to reading an excerpt from a fictional work, I would usually give a brief summary of a short story or a novel to present an excerpt within the wider context. Handouts with reading materials were distributed to the group at the beginning of each session. Specific criteria for selecting materials included:

- relevance of materials to the topics addressed
- high literary quality of fiction and poetry
- evidence-based support for non-fiction materials
- the diversity of cultural and spiritual traditions reflected in readings.

I have ensured the high quality of reading materials by selecting fiction and poetry by prominent classical and contemporary authors. When selecting non-fictional materials (e.g. works in psychology, philosophy, environmental sciences, neuroscience), I considered the author's expertise in a particular field and focused on including renowned authors in different fields of the humanities, sciences and social sciences (Table 5.1).

Table 5.1 *Examples of fiction, non-fiction and poetry authors used in Read to Connect*

Fiction authors	Non-fiction authors	Poets
Paul Bowles		Robert Frost
Joseph Boyden	Norman Doidge	Mary Oliver
Ivan Bunin	Leo Buscaglia	Lord Byron
Paolo Coelho	Victor Frankl	Rainer Maria Rilke
Kate Chopin	Thich Nhat Hanh	Percy Shelley
Charles Dickens	Erich Fromm	John Clare
Elizabeth Hay	Jean-Paul Sartre	Juan Ramon Jimenez
Ernest Hemingway	Jean Vanier	Kobayashi Issa
Hermann Hesse	Jon Kabat-Zinn	Leonard Cohen
Alistair MacLeod	Dalai Lama	Chief Dan George
Toni Morrison		Rumi
Alice Munro	Andrey Tarkovsky	Alexander Pushkin
Vladimir Nabokov		Shakespeare
Ben Okri	Elizabeth Kubler-Ross	James Kavanaugh
Antoine de Saint-Exupery	David Suzuki	Emily Dickinson
Leo Tolstoy	Thomas Berry	Rabindranath Tagore
William P. Young		Shel Silverstein

The use of poetry has proved to be especially beneficial in triggering quick responses that would engage the group in meaningful discussions. A wide variety of poems included into thematic compilations represented different poetic traditions and styles: Japanese haiku masters; Persian, English, Russian, Indian, European and American classics; Native American poets; and contemporary European, American and Canadian poets. At the beginning of the programme many participants admitted that they did not like poetry, but they later volunteered to read the poems aloud and connected well to the poems included into compilations. The communication around poetic pieces provided good examples in support for the notion that in bibliotherapy 'the individual's feeling-response is more important than an intellectual grasp of the work's meaning' (Hynes and Hynes-Berry, 1986, 43). Without contemplating the whole poem in the complexity of its themes and stylistic features, participants would often connect to one line and share reflection, a memory or a personal story triggered by this line. They would often enter the discussion with phrases like: 'I agree with what he says here;' 'I disagree;' 'this is true;' 'I feel the same;' or 'I like how he says.' One of the participants expressed his appreciation of the poems included in compilations and provided a powerful argument in support for the use of poetry during the reading sessions: 'this is about life.'

Considering the diversity of the group, the goal was to select the readings that would speak to individuals representing different cultural and spiritual traditions. This is particularly important when working with the diverse population of Toronto, where multiculturalism and diversity are the key characteristics of the client groups participating in local community programmes and services. Given the flexibility in selecting materials for a reading session, it was always possible to include readings that would meet the interests of a diverse group. For example, the materials included into the compilation *Connecting to Nature* included poems by Emily Dickinson; Native American poems and songs; Japanese haikus; excerpts from the novel *The Old Man and the Sea* by Ernest Hemingway; excerpts from the environmental works by David Suzuki and Thomas Berry; and excerpts from writings by the Dalai Lama.

Due to the walk-in format of weekly reading sessions, the programme's design did not include a formal evaluation. However, the participants were asked to fill out the questionnaire at the end of the programme. The participants' feedback provided through informal conversations and completed evaluation forms showed that the programme created a warm and welcoming environment for reading 'good books', 'talking about life' and sharing personal stories. Some acknowledged that they were looking forward to the Friday sessions and revisiting the readings at home. Participants highlighted the programme features that particularly appealed to them, such as reading aloud, the variety of materials included into compilations, the length of reading materials and the opportunity to meet people and share their stories. They also expressed appreciation for the passion and the courage of the facilitator:

> You are a brave woman reading children's books to us [referring to *The Giving Tree*, by Shel Silverstein] but I liked it.

The charity's staff also found the programme to be beneficial and perceived it as a valuable addition to available support services.

While closely observing the participants' response to readings articulated in their reflections, I have captured many consoling, if not therapeutic, moments experienced by those who found similarity between the stories read or told during the sessions and their personal life experiences. The interactions between the texts and the group provided examples of a common literary response in bibliotherapy known as *universalization* – the 'recognition that you are not the only one who feels a certain way' (Brewster, 2009, 14). During the discussions around the fictional or real-life challenges portrayed in the books – whether it was a story of relocation, destructive family relationships, unfulfilled love or betrayal – the participants would often acknowledge the fact that they struggled with similar issues in their past or present life situations. The meaning collectively constructed through creative interaction around the texts would not only provide insights into the nature of addressed 'problems of living' in general, but stimulated a sense of shared fate. The latter, as reflected in one of the participant's remarks – 'it helps to know that you are not all alone' – helped dispel feelings of loneliness and isolation. As Gold (1990, 47) asserts, 'being recognized by the book' can have a strong consoling effect on a reader: it makes them feel less alone and more 'normal'. This resonates with the observation by Simon du Plock (2005, 305) who suggests that for clients in bibliotherapy, literature has 'the function of raising awareness and providing a sense of connectedness to a community of suffering, or more broadly, a community of experience'. Given the fact that the majority of existing life problems of a personal or social nature have been addressed through world literature multiple times and from multiple perspectives, this notion has an important implication for bibliotherapy.

On many occasions, the participants demonstrated empathy and compassion when listening to both fictional stories and those shared by the group members. One particularly powerful moment took place during the reading session on forgiveness. Following the reading from the novel *The Shack*, by William Paul Young, one of the group members shared a story describing his personal journey from feelings of hatred and thoughts of revenge to the full forgiveness of the individual who caused him a severe emotional pain. After a moment of deep silence, the group exploded in words of support, empathy and appreciation of his experience. They also expressed gratitude to him for sharing this story with the group. These moments would build trust and reinforce the willingness to share – a powerful way of restoring connections with the world and people around. This observation supports the findings of studies that emphasize the importance of reading and communication around the texts in building a sense of community among people with similar problems (Billington et al., 2010; Davis et al., 2012; Hodge, Robinson and Davis, 2007).

Overall, the observations made throughout the programme implementation showed that creative interaction with literary texts, enhanced by the unifying power of a reading group discussion, may have a transformational effect on individuals involved in this activity. By connecting to stories in the books and those shared by reading group members, individuals can not only rewrite their own narratives, but also live through situations that they may never have a chance to encounter in their lives. The latter can be especially beneficial for those who are trapped within life situations that they are not able to change (for example, individuals affected by a chronic illness or disability) or those dealing with stigmatization. The realization that I have facilitated some positive change by connecting books and people that otherwise would never have met was one of the most rewarding moments for me as a facilitator.

Further development: the Bibliotherapy for Staff programme

Given the flexibility of the described bibliotherapy approach with regards to both theme and material selection, it was possible to easily adjust it to the needs of a different client group. In 2012, I launched the Bibliotherapy for Staff programme for the staff of the Scarborough and Rouge Hospital (formerly Rouge Valley Health System) in Toronto. Within the context of traditional workplace wellness programmes and services, the bibliotherapy-based library programme aimed to provide a new venue to address workplace wellness and promote a healthy lifestyle to hospital employees. It was implemented in collaboration with the staff of the Occupational Health department, who participated in theme selection and helped promote the service within the organization. The targeted population included both clinical and non-clinical groups, including nurses, physicians, allied health professionals and the hospital administration. A detailed description of the programme, outlining its mechanics, benefits and challenges is available elsewhere (Tukhareli, 2017).

The thematic compilations of readings addressed core existential themes (e.g. resilience, power of gratitude, purpose in life, gift of love) and more specific work-related issues (such as life–work balance, meaningful work, work stress and change management), thus providing the programme participants with an opportunity to get insight into their own situations in life and at work. The reading materials were selected from a broad variety of both fiction and non-fiction texts. However, unlike the Read to Connect programme, the compilations included a larger volume of non-fiction materials. While fiction and poetry provided a chance for reflection and observation, non-fiction materials educated staff on resilience-building strategies supported by recent developments in the fields of positive psychology, neuroplasticity and complementary therapies. The compilations included excerpts from the evidence-based articles retrieved from biomedical databases (Medline/PubMed), online magazines (*Greater Good Magazine*; *Psychology Today*; HealthGuide.org) and non-fiction texts. Example texts used in Bibliotherapy for Staff include:

- Elaine Fox (2012) *Rainy Brain, Sunny Brain: how to retrain your brain to overcome pessimism and achieve a more positive outlook*
- Victor Strecher (2016) *Life on Purpose: how living for what matters most changes everything*
- Elena Mannes (2011) *The Power of Music: pioneering discoveries in the new science of song*
- Robert A. Emmons (2007) *Thanks! How the New Science of Gratitude Can Make You Happier*
- Norman Doidge (2015) *The Brain's Way of Healing: remarkable discoveries and recoveries from the frontiers of neuroplasticity*
- Jon Kabat-Zinn (2006) *Coming to Our Senses: healing ourselves and the world through mindfulness*
- Rick Hanson (2013) *Hardwiring Happiness: the new brain science of contentment, calm, and confidence.*

The compilations of readings were delivered to staff through the library's website, a weekly hospital electronic newsletter and customized e-mails to specific clinical groups.

The programme evaluation included an internal survey to the hospital employees. We were particularly interested in the participants' responses to the following statements:

- Readings contributed to improved wellbeing (provided relaxation and/or reduced stress).

- Readings provided insights or a new perspective on my current situation in life and/or at work.

Twenty-six out of 32 respondents rated both statements between seven and ten (on a scale of one to ten, with ten being the highest). Respondents also expressed their overall satisfaction with the variety and quality of materials selected (28 out of 32) and the length of compilations (27 out of 32). Overall, the programme has been recognized as an effective way of addressing workplace wellness within a hospital environment. From the hospital library's perspective, it has expanded opportunities for collaborative projects and increased visibility of the library within the organization.

The success of shared reading groups expanding across the UK and internationally and the demonstrated potential of the bibliotherapy approach featured in Read to Connect and Bibliotherapy for Staff programmes have motivated me to advocate the further development and promotion of creative bibliotherapy in Canada. Raising the profile of creative bibliotherapy through publications, conference presentations and media interviews disseminating the benefits of the creative bibliotherapy approach has led to other organizations integrating it into their programmes and services. In the autumn of 2015, I co-facilitated a reading programme for the clients of the STAR (Supporting Transitions and Recovery) Learning Centre, an adult education programme for homeless people at St Michael's Hospital in Toronto. In 2017, two pilot projects were launched in the province of Ontario: a reading programme for the clients of the Ontario Shores Centre for Mental Health Sciences in Whitby and a programme run by the owner of an independent book store in collaboration with a local health authority in Waterloo. I hope that in the future, the facilitators of these reading projects will document more successful stories of how books can guide, console and even change one's life.

Conclusion

Overall, the findings of the bibliotherapy programmes described in this chapter supported the previously published evidence that creative bibliotherapy, in a variety of its clinical and non-clinical applications, provides a safe and inspirational venue for self-exploration and social relationships. Within the context of the increased focus on personal growth and social inclusion in approaches to mental health, bibliotherapy-based reading programmes provide a cost-effective, accessible and creative way of helping individuals cope with the challenges of everyday life. Recent qualitative and quantitative evidence suggests a variety of psychological and social benefits for the participants of these programmes.

Considering the flexibility of the described bibliotherapy approach in addressing the needs of various population groups, I believe that it has potential for future development. I suggest that it should be further explored within a framework of traditional support groups that are run by peer group leaders or professionals within clinical and community settings, as well as the stress-management and wellness programmes offered at workplaces. Describing a positive impact of support groups on their participants, Adamsen (2002, 224) asserts: 'it is evident that the positive effects of self-help groups are mainly because of their inherent capacity for universalizing personal problems'. Taking into consideration that universalization is known as a key element of success of bibliotherapy, I would argue that the integration of fiction, poetry and non-fiction (biographies, autobiographies and memoirs) in a traditional support or wellness group structure can provide its participants with more opportunities for universalization and comparison, thus significantly expanding therapeutic space for clients. On the other hand, the use of informational and self-help resource materials can help promote healthy living tools and resilience-building strategies within the groups. The latter is particularly important when working with individuals who are limited in their ability to access high-quality consumer health and self-help books, websites and other resources.

Finally, I share the belief that creative bibliotherapy can fill a unique niche within the context of services and programmes traditionally offered in a hospital or public library setting (Brewster, 2008). In this regard, I also encourage librarians to better utilize their literary knowledge and critical appraisal skills by getting actively engaged in finding new creative ways of connecting great literature and evidence-based informational resources with individuals who are left behind by traditional book clubs and health information workshops run in the libraries. As for the librarians' ethical concerns about overstepping their professional boundaries and getting involved in therapy, one way to overcome this barrier is by collaborating with healthcare and social service providers (psychologists, counsellors and social workers) when integrating bibliotherapy into a library setting. Overall, bibliotherapy opens new opportunities for partnership and collaboration for both public and medical libraries, which fits into their agenda to expand the list of outreach services offered to local communities.

Dedication

This chapter is dedicated to the memory of Joseph Gold, whose insights into the nature and benefits of bibliotherapy have inspired me on my own journey in the field.

References

Adamsen, L. (2002) 'From Victim to Agent': the clinical and social significance of self-help group participation for people with life-threatening diseases, *Scandinavian Journal of Caring Sciences*, **16** (3), 224–31.

Billington, J., Dowrick, C., Hamer, A., Robinson, J. and Williams, C. (2010) *An Investigation into Therapeutic Benefits of Reading in Relation to Depression and Wellbeing*, LivHIR Research Report.

Billington, J., Jones, A., Humphreys, A. L. and McDonnell, K. (2014) *An Evaluation of a Literature-Based Intervention for People with Chronic Pain*, LivHIR Research Report.

Brewster, L. (2008). The Reading Remedy: bibliotherapy in practice. *Australian Public Libraries and Information Services*, **21** (4), 172–7.

Brewster, L. (2009). Reader Development and Mental Wellbeing: the accidental bibliotherapist, *Australian Public Libraries and Information Services*, **22** (1), 13–16.

Carty, S., Thompson, L., Berger, S., Jahnke, K. and Llewellyn R. (2016) Books on Prescription – Community Based Health Initiative to Increase Access to Mental Health Treatment: an evaluation, *Australian and New Zealand Journal of Public Health*, **40** (3), 276–8.

Cheu, H. (2001) There is No Class in this Text: from reader-response to bibliotherapy, *Textual Studies in Canada*, **13/14** (Summer), 37–46.

Davis J. (2009) Enjoying and Enduring: groups reading aloud for wellbeing, *Lancet*, **373** (9665), 714–15.

Davis, J. (2017) Literature isn't a Luxury but a Life-changer. *The Guardian*, (2 April), www.theguardian.com/commentisfree/2017/apr/01/reading-organization-shared-education-wider-audience.

Davis, P., Billington, J., Carroll, J., Healey, C. and Kinderman, P. (2012) *A Literature-based Intervention for Older People Living with Dementia*, LivHIR Research Report.

Doidge, N. (2007) *The Brain that Changes Itself: stories of personal triumph from the frontiers of brain science*, Penguin Books.

Dowrick, C., Billington, J., Robinson J., Hamer, A. and Williams, C. (2012) Get into Reading as an Intervention for Common Mental Health Problems: exploring catalysts for change. *Medical Humanities*, **38** (1), 15–20.

Du Plock, S. (2005). 'Silent therapists' and 'the community of suffering', *Existential Analysis*, **16** (2), 300–9.

Gold, J. (1990) *Read for Your Life: literature as a life support system*, Fitzhenry & Whiteside.

Gold, J. (2002) *The Story Species: our life-literature connection*, Fitzhenry & Whiteside.

Hodge, S., Robinson, J. and Davis, P. (2007) Reading Between the Lines: the experiences of taking part in a community reading project, *Journal of Medical Ethics*, **33**, 100–4.

Hynes, A. M. and Hynes-Berry, M. (1986) *Bibliotherapy. The Interactive Process: a handbook*, Westview Press.

MacLeod, A. (2000) *Island: the collected stories*, McClelland & Steward.

Mendel, M. R., Harris, J. and Carson, N. (2016) Bringing Bibliotherapy for Children to Clinical Practice, *Journal of the American Academy of Child & Adolescent Psychiatry*, **55** (7), 535–7.

Oatley, K. (1999) Meetings of Minds: dialogue, sympathy, and identification in reading fiction, *Poetics*, **26**, 439–54.

Rilke, R. M. (2011) Letters to a Young Poet (translated and edited by C. Louth), Penguin.

Robertson, J. and Billington, J. (2013) *An Evaluation of a Pilot Study of a Literature-Based Intervention with Women in Prison*, LivHIR Research Report.

Robertson, R., Wray, S. J., Maxwell, M. and Pratt, R. J. (2008) The Introduction of a Healthy Reading Scheme for People with Mental Health Problems: usage and experiences of health professionals and library staff, *Mental Health in Family Medicine*, **5**, 219–28.

Robinson, J. (2008a) *Reading and Talking: exploring the experience of taking part in reading groups at the Walton Neuro-Rehabilitation Unit (NRU)*, HaCCRU Research Report, 114/08.

Robinson, J. (2008b) *Reading and Talking: exploring the experience of taking part in reading groups at the Vauxhall Health Care Centre*, HaCCRU Research Report, 115.

Tukhareli, N. (2011) Bibliotherapy in a Library Setting: reaching out to vulnerable youth, *The Canadian Journal of Library and Information Practice and Research*, **6** (1), 1–18.

Tukhareli, N. (2014) *Healing through Books: the evolution and diversification of bibliotherapy*, Edwin Mellen Press.

Tukhareli, N. (2017) Bibliotherapy-based Wellness Program for Healthcare Providers: using books and reading to create a healthy workplace, *Journal of the Canadian Health Libraries Association/Journal de l'Association des bibliothèques de la santé du Canada*, **38**, 44–50.

Volpe, U., Torre, F., De Santis, V., Perris, F. and Catapano, F. (2015) Reading Group Rehabilitation for Patients with Psychosis: a randomized controlled study, *Clinical Psychology & Psychotherapy*, **22**, 15–21.

Walsh, T. (2010) The Power of Words, *Nursing Standard*, **24** (49), 20–1.

6

Long-term impacts of bibliotherapy groups: reading and writing together

Fiona Bailey

Introduction

Braw Blether[1] – a Book Group With a Difference promises 'there is no preparation required'. Removing the pressure to read a book you have not chosen has been proven to engage individuals looking for a different way into reading. Since the onset, these weekly, library-based sessions, using words for wellbeing, have witnessed long-term attendance.

When I began the role of Healthy Reading Bibliotherapist, the service was entering its third year and had retained a number of original group members. I have been continually struck by the level of commitment they display. Each week, I observe the group arriving, often carrying books or photographs from home that in some way follow on from the previous week's conversation. Participants can face an eventful morning: some rely on assisted transport, others wait indoors for a support worker to help with the morning routine. Occasionally, people arrive in suits from a job interview, other times a funeral – yet attending the group remains an obvious priority.

External and ongoing internal evaluations have shown multiple benefits to participants' health and wellbeing, including increased relaxation, improved confidence and escapism, all possible from a single session. However, further qualitative data from recent case studies highlighted some longer-term outcomes, namely a continued passion for reading and sharing of books; a growing sense of community for previously isolated individuals; and a rise in confidence resulting in emerging creative work.

This chapter reflects on the advantages and ongoing challenges of bibliotherapy work without a clear ending. Through reflection on my first year as a new facilitator to two well established bibliotherapy groups, I explore ways of maintaining a healthy group dynamic over time. This includes the selection of session material; developing trust and group cohesion; supporting creativity; and addressing issues around stigma. The chapter concludes with a set of practical tips based on my experiences managing the challenges of facilitating a long-standing bibliotherapy service.

Background to the bibliotherapy service

Midlothian, located to the south of Edinburgh, experiences considerable socio-economic disparity: some of the most expensive properties in Scotland co-exist with areas of high unemployment and deprivation stemming largely from the long-term decline of the traditional local mining industry. The library services perform a vital social inclusion, regeneration and lifelong learning role in communities. Of some 88,000 Midlothian inhabitants, more than 28,000 (almost one in three) have a library card.

Midlothian Libraries' Bibliotherapy service was set up in 2014 and has three regular library-based groups. Funding in 2014 was provided by the Scottish Libraries and Information Council Public Libraries Improvement Fund and was initially perceived as a 'next step' beyond the Books on Prescription scheme. Funding for years two and three came from the Integrated Care Fund, a local source using health and social care integration money from the Scottish Government. The service holds an extensive 'toolkit' or resource built from externally funded outreach projects tailored to specific client groups. Settings include a recovery café for individuals affected by addictions; secondary schools; and a collaboration with a service supporting young people excluded from mainstream education.

There are two core weekly groups – one based at Dalkeith Library (with an average of three to five participants) and the other based at Penicuik Library (with an average of five to nine participants). Braw Blether is advertised widely, attracting participants with wide-ranging needs and abilities. Promotional material deliberately targets individuals with poor mental health and wellbeing, but offers the individual the choice whether they wish to openly identify with a mental health difficulty or not. Many participants find Braw Blether through word of mouth, often at the recommendation of library staff; others discover the group via a GP, occupational therapist or organizations such as the Red Cross. Participants of Braw Blether need not be library members.

There is also a monthly Braw Blether for Carers group which has six regular members. This all-female group met through a local organization supporting full-time carers in 2013 and in 2016 encountered a 'taster' session with the Healthy Reading Bibliotherapist. The group tend to rate the benefits of bibliotherapy similarly to the two core groups, but prefer not to have a group agreement and adopt a more relaxed approach to facilitation. In summary, the group report that Braw Blether for Carers has strengthened their existing friendships, provided much needed escapism from the caring role, and broadened reading horizons.

Development of the current bibliotherapy provision

As a new facilitator to well-established groups, I considered what benefits and challenges my own background would bring to the current working model. Studying Creative Writing had led me into bibliotherapy work, but my background in group facilitation was mainly through nursing, counselling and a specialist liaison post in the National Health Service (NHS). The main difference with Braw Blether was the wide range of backgrounds of participants, coupled with the fact that there is no openly shared experience between members, such as loss.

In keeping with the non-clinical space, Midlothian Libraries use a social, rather than medical, bibliotherapy model. The non-clinical spaces I had been used to previously were empty offices overlooking city hospitals or recently vacated patient side rooms with the broken equipment piled down one end. In contrast, the library setting provides a sense of freedom and promotes a sense of wellness in the absence of medical professionals. As one member put it:

> Libraries are quite a welcoming place; they're neutral territory . . . it doesn't feel like it's the school's, the school kids' or anybody else's.

The use of imaginative texts, rather than self-help literature, helps achieve the desired escapism. I was keen to model the group agreement as a way of building trust, acknowledging both groups' requests for fun or escapism and meeting it with carefully selected material.

With the wide-ranging needs of the participants in mind, ongoing professional development for the Healthy Reading Bibliotherapist is supported through clinical supervision within the council's Social Work department. Further to this, a steering group, including a psychological psychotherapist, Child and Adolescent Mental Health Services (CAMHS) and a joint mental health officer from the local authority, meet regularly to help guide the service delivery.

Using the evaluation tool as a starting point

When I took over responsibility for the groups in August 2016, Braw Blether was approaching the start its third year and, I was keen to ensure all was working well. As a new facilitator, it was helpful to think of the outcomes from previous evaluations and to consider opportunities for building trust. The main evaluation tool used by the service is called, 'What has biblio-therapy helped you do?'. It lists ten outcomes for participants to rate in effectiveness from 1 to 4 (see Figure 6.1). This is used by the bibliotherapist every few months.

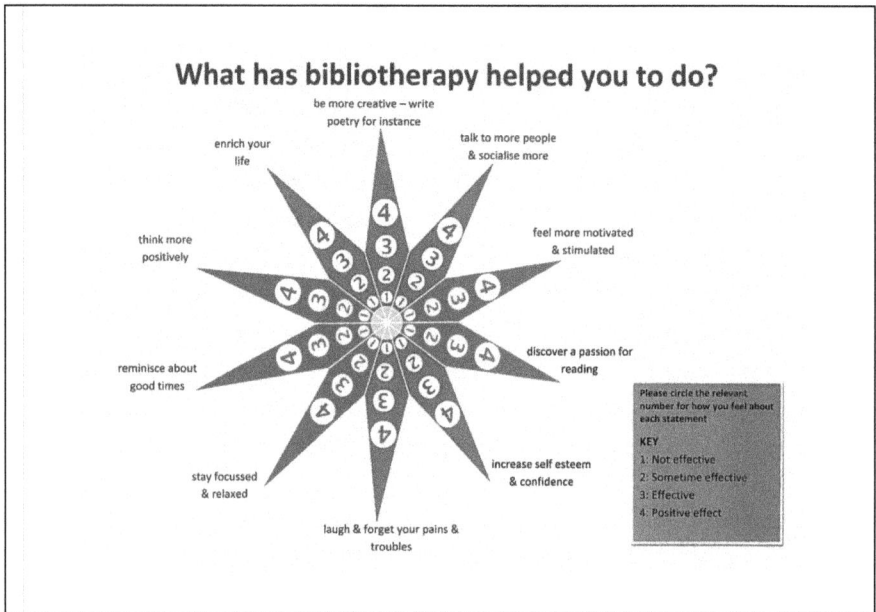

Figure 6.1 *The Outcome Star, based on the tool used by Kirklees Council and Camden, Westminster and Derbyshire local authorities in the UK*

In 2016, these outcomes formed part of an external evaluation in which sixteen people participated. A few participants went on to take part in semi-structured interviews, forming case studies, while others took part in a focus group. Figure 6.2 opposite shows the average ratings for each statement on the star evaluation. All ten statements were rated above average or higher by both groups, with 'socializing', 'motivation and stimulation', and 'enrich your life' rated most highly.

From the ten outcomes, 'laugh and forget your pains and troubles', 'stay focused and relaxed' and 'reminisce about good times' seem to tie in with escapism, so this seemed a sensible theme to consider in early session planning.

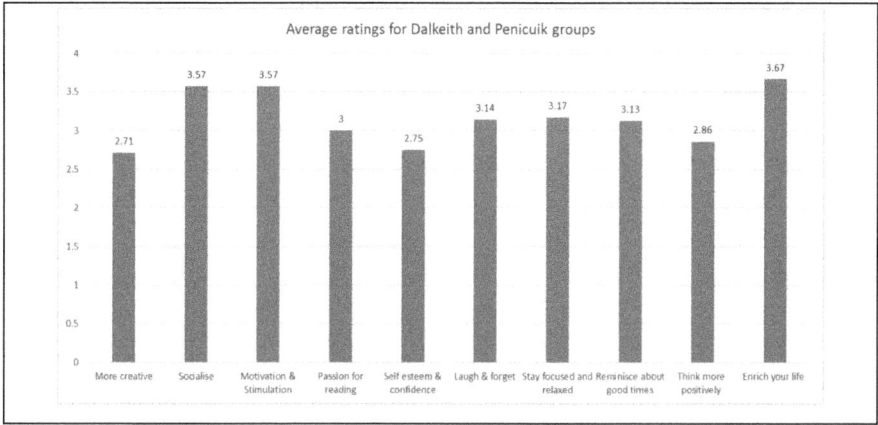

Figure 6.2   *Average ratings across the two groups for the Outcome Star evaluations.*

Selecting material to build trust

Escapism, I quickly learned, often came in the form of crime fiction, especially for the group at Dalkeith Library. A page-turner was the best way to unwind, the bloodier the better. The most borrowed titles were from Ian Rankin and Ann Cleeves. Keen to follow the group's interests, but restricted by the 90-minute session, I eventually decided on a collection of Murder Ballads. One participant struggled to concentrate beyond about 150 words at a time. The group had also expressed a disinterest in poetry, which presented a further challenge.

We began with 17th-century folklore, 'Twa' Sisters', moving on to Tom Waits' version. Last of all, we read Bob Dylan's 'Hurricane'. The group were particularly struck by the true story of the false imprisonment of Rubin 'Hurricane' Carter. Participants recounted their favourite, flawed, fictional detectives and admitted a few similar traits of their own. The group discussed the ways murder ballads either focused on jealousy, as in crimes of passion, or protest songs as a result of injustice.

These early sessions helped me identify themes that were particularly helpful to spark conversation with both groups, such as injustice. Another useful piece of material came from a *New Yorker* article called 'The Encyclopedia Reader' (Gross, 2016): a tale of a metaphorical escape through learning to read with a prison library service. This true story tapped into a renewed enjoyment of crime biographies and also uncovered a few reading 'demons' from people's early years. As we learn how Woods, the prisoner, is excluded from the classroom growing up, the group shared some of their early reading experiences: growing up in houses without books or encountering an unwritten hierarchy of reading material. This gave me some insight into attitudes towards poetry: it was seen in some households as frivolous and in some classrooms as purely for critique.

An additional challenge in addressing the needs of these long-term groups is that there is no one-size-fits-all approach. At Christmas, rather than gathering festive material to make use of the seasonal prompts, I asked the group about their attitudes to Christmas and New Year, which it turned out differed greatly. One group found December a difficult month and made a survival guide for the holidays. It proved helpful to consider what support others might need at Christmas. Another group cut out text from Christmas carols to make an alternative reading.

The weekly challenge of finding engaging material meant that I was keen to find ways to reintroduce poetry more regularly, emphasizing to the group there was no need to critique the poems. With this in mind, I asked the group if 'there's no need to critique the material' would be a useful addition to the group agreement. It was fortunate timing that November 2016 saw the launch of Brian Bilston's crowdfunded poetry collection following his rise to fame on social media. His poems are ideal in length – many are tweets – and deceptively simple, often requiring a second reading. Bilston's (2016) work contains refreshingly mundane subject matter: bin day or the perils of trying to fold a fitted sheet. The universal struggles with day-to-day life proved a useful bonding tool for the group. 'Refugees', which can be read forwards or backwards, literally turned reading poetry on its head. Poems such as 'Grammar Police' shine a light on poetry snobs and play with form – which provided a useful gateway to creative writing exercises later on.

Developing trust and group cohesion

A few months into the post, I noticed trust had developed enough for one or two participants to hint at the unacknowledged reasons that led them to join the group. Due to the openness of the referrals and a gap in the service before I arrived, I knew very little about individual reasons for coming. When the group expressed a surprise at this, it was a useful reminder that I had missed the first two years of an ongoing conversation and that there was an opportunity to retell some stories. This progression came as a relief to me as this lack of disclosure had made planning the sessions with fun and escapism in mind an increasing challenge.

The existing group agreement mentioned that personal issues might get in the way of an enjoyable group experience and there were some things best saved until the group had finished. It also stated 'avoid talking about the past too much' and 'reminisce about good times'. The agreement had been used to address some quite specific issues which were no longer relevant and I had reached a point where it felt impossible to select material that would not trigger the ever-present past. Revisiting the group agreement went a long way to enable me to work with different levels of disclosure. To manage unavoidable triggers each week, I also asked the group to consider what happens if something we read or hear feels difficult. The group agreed to add a statement 'Everyone has the right to "pass"'. This complemented the original agreement that there was no pressure to share.

On the subject of unintended consequences arising from material for therapeutic purposes: Bowman (2004) suggests considering your desired outcome and how it will affect the direction of the group, asking yourself 'What's the worst that could happen?'. With this in mind, I took along a handful of printed portraits of poets with known or suspected mental illness, enough so that each member of the group could take one and read a short paragraph which included a struggle in the poet's life. Then we read an accompanying poem from their legacy.

When we had finished reading John Clare's poem *I Am*, people immediately returned to the first line, 'I am – yet what I am none cares or knows'. Where previous invitations to respond to a poem had fallen a little flat, this line was read repeatedly. The group quickly found common ground in the stigma attached to mental illness, and often in creativity. Struck by the date of the poem from 1748 and how relevant the first line felt, people speculated at how their own struggles might have been perceived over 250 years ago. Two individuals who are wheelchair users talked about current attitudes to disability, acknowledging that the invisible struggles, such as depression and anxiety, were sometimes more difficult to manage. There were further disclosures: one about a recent in-patient stay in a local psychiatric hospital, another about bullying in the workplace leading to a forced resignation. All agreed that individuals have a right to be known. Through the poet's experience of stigma, similar experiences were shared. Often one story gives permission to tell another.

I was left wondering about the long-term impact this obvious shift in the nature of group discussion might bring about. As the group had shared memories of an abandoned Victorian asylum nearby, the following week I took a few photographs from the local history archive. My intention was to offer some continuity, whilst shifting the focus onto the surrounding landscape by introducing one or two nature poems from a local writer. The feeling on returning was positive. Individuals had taken a risk in disclosing personal insight, but seemed to feel there was permission to move in another direction with the change in material. This session was lighter. I had also underestimated the influence of the changing setting in the library from week to week. In this case, both the setting and the text helped to 'reset' the balance.

There have been a number of unexpected longer-term outcomes of this ongoing bibliotherapy work. Firstly, there is an increased sense of community through ongoing mutual support. The group members are frequently promoting the group locally, including one member who has a regular feature on a local radio station. Furthermore, bibliotherapy groups can be a gateway to other groups, including more traditional reading and writing groups. People reported using other local facilities, like the gym, when going to and from Braw Blether. Another notable outcome is participants' immense pride in the perceived success of the group and the interest from local press and further afield, including BBC Radio Scotland. Finally, a further outcome is the deepening of existing friendships. Over the longer term, confidence and self-worth have increased through the feeling of mutual support within the group.

Creative outputs

Although increased creativity scored the lowest amongst the measured outcomes during the evaluation (see Figure 6.2), there has been a great deal of written work produced within the core groups. The wording of the outcome star 'write poetry for instance' might have been misleading for some. The participants may well underestimate the level of creative output, as writing is deliberately not included in the groups' expectations or unwritten 'terms of engagement'. Attendees generally expect to 'blether' and to read aloud a little, but writing has always been an optional extra, reflecting the wide range of abilities the group invites. Therefore, as the facilitator of Braw Blether I do not rely too heavily on writing exercises.

It helps to call the writing 'expressive' rather than creative. Many participants have had bad experiences of writing at school or in creative writing groups. The group agreement also now states 'there's no such thing as good writing' and as a facilitator I encourage people to notice what is interesting in a piece of writing and what they want to know more about, rather than asking them to make a judgement about it. At one library, the group simply claps for each piece shared.

Of course, participants have the right to 'pass' on sharing work. Sometimes writing prompts have brought about an unexpected creation. On one occasion, a participant assembled four left-over words from a cut-up exercise, drawing my attention to them before sweeping them into the bin. It was positive for him to acknowledge the work. Another participant wrote down her mother's old shopping list from memory. With some persuasion she kept the piece, which now serves as a tool to invite nostalgia in other library groups.

Tackling stigma

An external evaluation in March 2017 by Blake Stevenson on behalf of the Public Library Improvement Fund focused on the long-term success of the weekly groups (Blake Stevenson Ltd, 2017). While Braw Blether participants again described the library as a neutral, familiar and comforting environment, one or two attendees reported feeling stigmatized. The case studies from the previous evaluation noted a stigma attached to attending a 'support group', despite it not being within a medical setting. For the participants preferring not to disclose any mental health difficulties, the library setting and the literary material can offer handy euphemisms. The name Braw Blether was chosen by the group members and it is used interchangeably with terms such as 'the book group' or 'the library group'. The issue of stigma being off-putting has begun to be reflected in the promotional material. Quotes from ongoing feedback from participants speak for themselves:

It opens up the world . . . you get to feel as though you're a world citizen again

It's what I look forward to all week

It does lead to curiosity about other books, it does broaden the mind, it does challenge your perceptions . . . it's gone a long way to conquering social anxiety . . . it's made me feel as if I've got a voice.

Challenges and considerations for long-term bibliotherapy work

Long-term bibliotherapy work offers stability to people with changing circumstances and provides security to explore issues. The journey through the library each week can be grounding. Changing scenery outside and displays within the library feeding into the time of year can help to restore perspective. One library has sessions beyond a glass partition. There are always interruptions, but babies tapping on the glass or someone knocking over a pile of books can bring life to a group session. The facilitator can encourage and nurture contributions from the group without pressurizing people to contribute. Knowing the group will meet regularly is useful for some. Yet working without a set ending can be overwhelming for others who are less likely to take risks in opening up indefinitely. Over a longer period, revisiting the group agreement gave me permission to ask the participants some bolder questions, such as 'What do you bring to the group?', thus gleaning more detail about the long-term mechanisms at play.

Some of the longer-term participants commented on the fact they would have personally found it hard to join an existing group. New people joining Braw Blether 'late' report there has been no awkwardness, but knowing the duration of the existing group can be off-putting for some. Changing material each week can make newcomers feel more included when they first attend. Long-term groups can form part of an individual's regular support network. Therefore, scheduling breaks and organizing appropriate cover or arranging good lines of communication in the event of a last-minute cancellation need strong consideration.

Library staff are an excellent source of referrals, using their relationships with customers to identify those who would benefit from bibliotherapy work. Awareness of the bibliotherapy groups among less experienced library staff, in turn, raises awareness of the diverse range of mental health issues people face. Library staff are also an obvious source of session material and there is potential to share material for similar library groups like reminiscence groups. However, it is important to emphasize that Midlothian Libraries deliberately avoid adding to work of library staff. The service is delivered wholly by a part-time Healthy Reading Bibliotherapist with the necessary specialist skills to facilitate and with the support of regular supervision and input from a multidisciplinary steering group.

Advice for facilitators

As a result of the experience of the Braw Blether groups, the following tips are suggested for facilitators of similar groups.

1 Consider how each session is opened. Deliberately not referring back to last week's session helps draws a line.

2 When the group has had a break, deliberately hang back while people congregate; sharing news can help people focus and settle before the facilitator arrives.

3 Never expect the same group twice – prepare for the unexpected.

4 Use existing group members to explain the group to newcomers; they always describe it best and usually offer a personal insight as part of the introduction.

5 Guests can bring life and allow retelling of stories. Guest facilitators might be volunteers wanting work experience or a member of the library staff.

6 Always have a back-up session prepared: a classic piece, something funny, a news article or a quote. These are sometimes useful to help end a session that has taken an unexpected turn.

7 Popular poems are so for a reason. Don't be afraid to use a piece more than once; there will be value in revisiting an old favourite.

8 For people struggling to get into reading or stuck in a rut, try looking for new context, for example, using cut-up techniques or grouping poems in an unusual way, by removing the titles for example.

Conclusion

This chapter suggests that groups with no set ending can have extremely positive outcomes for people, but these outcomes rely on ongoing sense-checking on the facilitator's part via ongoing review of the group agreement.

While qualitative data is valuable in bringing out unexpected benefits of long-term bibliotherapy work, it is important not to mistake resultant outcomes for goals or terms of engagement. Some participants will use the stability of a long-term group to make a transition to other group activities, further study or employment, while others will benefit from a regular support network.

There are of course advantages and ongoing challenges in facilitating a long-standing bibliotherapy service reflected in all bibliotherapy work. The key should be to set realistic expectations, and review and manage these throughout the process. The diversity within the modern library setting can have a strong impact on maintaining the balance of long-term work and can even manage to combat some of the stigma attached to groups for wellbeing by reframing the work in a literary context.

Notes

1 In Scots, 'braw' mean fine or pleasant and 'blether' means a lengthy chat
   between friends.

References

Bilston, B. (2016) *You Took the Last Bus Home.* Unpublished.

Blake Stevenson Ltd (2017) *Public Library Improvement Fund: evaluation of health-
   related projects final report,* Scottish Library and Information Council,
   https://scottishlibraries.org/media/1619/slic-plif-evaluation-final-report.pdf.

Bowman, T. (2004) Potential Misuses of Poetry Therapy: a process for reflecting on
   practice, *Journal of Poetry Therapy,* **16** (4), 223–30.

Gross, D. A. (2016) The Encyclopedia Reader, *The New Yorker,* 13 September,
   www.newyorker.com/books/page-turner/the-encyclopedia-reader.

7

The benefits of shared reading groups for those at risk of homelessness

Susan McLaine and Elizabeth Mackenzie

Introduction: bibliotherapy in the Australian context

An integral part of the evolution of bibliotherapy in Australia has been the development of partnerships with local organizations across sectors including community-aged care, residential-aged care, mental health, health, carers and public housing to deliver reading groups in community settings. Initial contact showed that local community-based service providers were attracted to the idea of branching out and working with others through a partnership with their local library. This chapter examines the role of collaborations in bibliotherapy focusing on a partnership developed between State Library Victoria and Prague House, a low-care residential facility of St Vincent's Hospital in Melbourne, Australia. Prague House offers specialized care in a home-like environment for its residents who mostly experience chronic mental illness and have backgrounds of homelessness. Prague House, as a low-care facility, offers residential support for people who still enjoy mobility and a degree of independence; their care needs are low, in contrast to people who require a high degree of assistance with mobility and personal care, and therefore a higher ratio of nursing and care staff.

At Prague House, a weekly reading group was introduced in 2010 and delivered by Susan McLaine, a leading advocate and provider of bibliotherapy in Australia. The reading group was facilitated by Susan along with Elizabeth Mackenzie, Prague House Activities and Wellbeing Programme Coordinator. Prague House is home to 45 male and female residents, many of whom have experienced homelessness or are at risk of it. Many of the residents experience chronic mental illness or have an alcohol-related acquired brain injury, and may have cognitive impairment as a consequence.

In planning the reading group, we took into account the routines of the care facility and scheduled the group around morning teatime, an unalterable ritual for residents living in this care facility. Approximately eight participants regularly attended the reading group each week, with others dropping in and out at times, depending on their health or as people entered or left the facility. Extra care was taken to provide fresh coffee and biscuits as familiar and comforting features of morning teatime, as well as a warm welcome and sense of inclusion. Taking the time to set up the room before the group members arrive provided seamless movement from coffee and biscuits to sitting down with the readings easily accessible from each chair. The setting provided a sense of the session being a private place in which people's ideas or thoughts are valued, as is each participant's presence. The start and end of the session provided opportunities for personal interactions to create a sense of belonging to help form the basis of safe relationships where trust is built.

In the reading programme, McLaine and Mackenzie discovered many areas in which the participants were seen to flourish as a result of using literature to foster change through therapeutic dialogue, and a sense of community through growing together through shared experience. The text introduced by the facilitator provided the main structure and focus for group discussion which referred to many life situations. The shared reading groups often assisted participants to change their beliefs and attitudes and contributed to the development of a more integrated sense of self, with increased self-awareness and acceptance. A special characteristic of bibliotherapy at Prague House has been the joy the group experienced in listening to the human voice, the literary form and each other, as well as the invitation to engage and play with the particular experience of literature. There is a definite sense of connectedness, belonging, safety and growth through being present in experience.

Being part of a reading group

Australian reading groups, such as this one at Prague House, have been inspired by the work of The Reader (www.thereader.org.uk), where participants listen to imaginative literature (fiction, inspirational stories and poetry) read aloud. The Reader is a UK charity responsible for pioneering the use of books and reading in therapeutic ways in community settings. Together, the facilitator and group members explore, contemplate and discuss their thoughts and feelings about the readings.

Many Prague House residents have experienced marginalization and stigma as a result of mental illness, brain injury and homelessness. The conditions of mental illness and of brain injury impose social isolation and marginalization within the broader community. Providing opportunities for social interaction and self-expression through taking part in the reading group was a goal of the programme. For such a diverse resident cohort, simply accepting the invitation to take part in a group was an important step and establishing the group was exciting and novel for participants and facilitators.

Reading groups have two distinct activities. In the first activity of listening, there is something about being read to that can assist in moving people into a more open and willing state of personal engagement. The second activity, the discussion, provides a moment where humans meet to engage in exploring their experiences and reflecting on their reality.

In reading groups, the listener can also be a reader. Each week copies of the story are offered to the participants as a way to provide a choice to follow along with the written word as well as the invitation to read aloud or to simply listen. In the early stages of the programme, it was reiterated each week that no one had to read aloud or join in the discussion unless they wished to. This approach provided the opportunity for the group members to be with other people without the pressure of an expectation to interact.

It was observed quite quickly that even though there was no pressure in the group for anyone to reveal more than they are comfortable with, group members often felt personally compelled to share. Because sharing related back to the narrative or the line of a poem, it provided a sense of safety and maintained focus. The group members are not just telling personal details or a random anecdote; instead their contribution reflects on the text. Reading in this way can assist readers to recognize themselves in, or otherwise relate to, a text and find insight through reflection.

Group members might share a reflection on their childhood and how a particular character's journey got them thinking about an event in their lives or may include some of their hopes for a particular character and hopes for their own future. There were times when people were brave enough in the group to reflect back on a time from their past and reveal that in retrospect they might have done things differently or taken the path of a particular character in the story.

Listening to the human voice, the literary form and each other

Little dog Algie began regularly arriving at Prague House. His owner, who lived down the street, was contacted each time using Algie's collar contact details. The owner eventually suggested that Algie had decided where he wanted to be, and Algie became a Prague House pet. Algie began to surprise us by appearing and staying during our sessions. This meant making his way up the stairs to the lounge room on the first floor, something he did not do often as he had a permanently damaged leg. During the sessions, at times he appeared to listen intently to the story along with everyone else.

On the day that the photograph in Figure 7.1 was taken, Algie had arrived on time for the start of the week's session, but one of the facilitators had been delayed and other participants had not arrived. Group members noticed Algie waiting at the door. While we were reconnecting over a warm drink, we pondered on how Algie remembered the day and time of the reading group. Algie's attendance in the group was more than his love of being with the people in the room; hearing the prosody of the human voice seemed to be as important to him as for the human listeners and he often looked up at the person reading.

Research indicates that dogs process speech, meaningful words and intonation in a similar way to humans, particularly when they are talked to

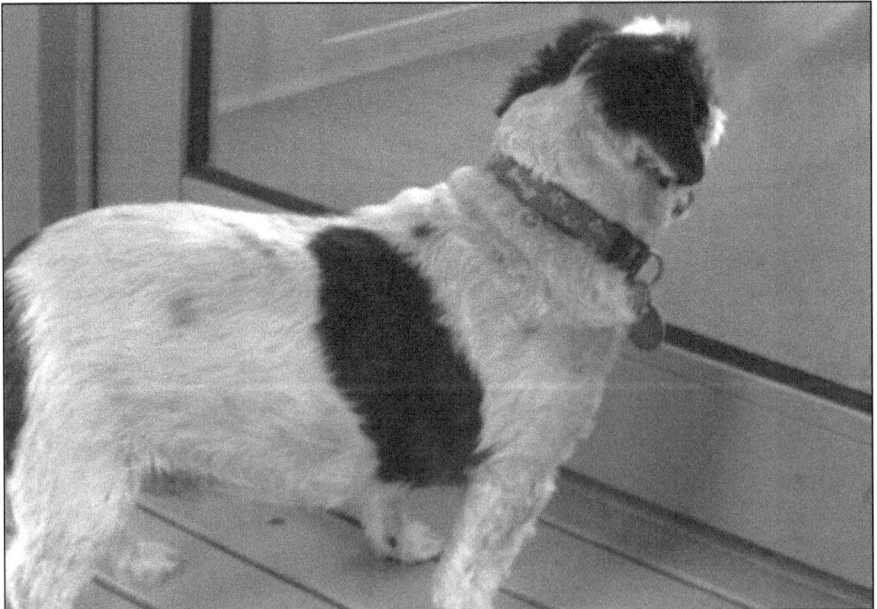

Figure 7.1 *Photograph of Algie, a Prague House pet*

on a regular basis (Radcliffe and Reby, 2014). People speak to babies and animals using exaggerated prosody (Jeannin et al., 2017), and living in a care environment, Algie was used to hearing praise words and intonation. Dogs use the same neural mechanisms as humans for language stimuli (left hemisphere) and for processing emotional tone sounds (right hemisphere) (Davis, 2016). It was evident that Algie was responding to emotional prosody in speech. 'There's something beautifully soothing about being read to' (Freeman-Greene, 2011) that contributes to the sense of safety in being part of a group for people feeling vulnerable in their isolation. Algie probably sensed how calm, relaxed and at ease his human friends were. This willingness to receive the words read aloud and the depth of listening was equally palpable in the engaged, quiet focus of the reading group.

Writers and poets select words for their sound as well as their meaning. The patterns of rhythm and sound of these words read aloud is referred to as 'prosody'. While prosody can be both verbal and non-verbal (Mitchell and Ross, 2013), and although several different types of prosody can be distinguished, emotional prosody is responsible for creating emotional tone and more subtle grades of meaning. Skidmore and Murakami (2016, 4) state that prosody includes the 'implicit readership of a written text that might have been set down centuries ago by an unknown hand.'

While bibliotherapy facilitators do not need to be trained in linguistics, they do need to have some knowledge of sound as a technical device when speaking. Using the key elements of intonation, volume and temporal occurrences such as rhythm, tempo, placement of stresses in a sentence and pauses ensures the effectiveness of the spoken piece. These elements influence the meaning of words and sentences to assist the group members to recognize the intention of the writer and to feel intimate with the distant voice of the writer (Hughes and Szczepek Reed, 2017; Mitchell and Ross, 2013).

The Prague House reading group members' health issues included dementia, brain damage, memory loss, hearing loss, schizophrenia and intellectual disabilities, in addition to cognitive impairment as a consequence of the impact of chronic mental illness or brain injury. For this particular group, it was essential to prepare the text to be read aloud by developing a sensitivity to the words, structure and poetic flow of the text. Understanding the effect of reading aloud, and how it supports the brain, language functions and processing of emotional cues, was a valuable resource to bring to the group. One of the group members expressed the importance of understanding the effect reading aloud can have; on hearing the words of a poem, Maurice said 'I can't make any sense of that!'. Maurice had had a recent exacerbation of his alcohol-related brain injury, to the extent that it was feared he had lost his ability to use language and a move to a higher-level care facility was being considered. He was struggling for words, but next he said, 'Something sinister must have been coming there'. We immediately saw that he was right – that the poem gave a metaphoric image of impending war.

An invitation to engage

Prose and poetry have an essential difference to that of ordinary language, no matter how similar to conversational language the text may at first seem to be (Oliver, 1994). It is important to provide leadership to the group by managing the space between literature and conversation through establishing the important boundary marker between the different activities of listening and discussion involved in reading groups. At the same time, an awareness of the non-verbal prosody within the group is needed; this has been described as simultaneously reading both the text and the group members. Being aware of the non-verbal prosody of the group members to support the rhythm and pace of the dialogue helps to create a connected and meaningful conversation.

Another group member, Colin, suffered from an intellectual disability as well as mental illness. Like many others experiencing chronic mental illness or brain injury he was withdrawn and shy and it took much courage to make his way upstairs each week to attend the group. When Colin was given a clear cue that we had finished listening to the story part of the session, he would indicate he was engaged by making sudden movements and lifting his head. Recently, after listening to a story featuring a beach, Colin's smile and expression glowed as he spoke of a childhood beach he remembered. Colin spent the rest of his time in the group relaxed in his chair with a smile on his face.

The writer's voice is heard, and their art is re-created, through reading aloud. It then becomes the creative object to which we respond and return, while listening to each other, finding our own truths. Winnicott (2005) writes of the therapeutic creative or 'play' space between individuals and literature. From the perspective of a facilitator, it is a constant delight to share participants' responses to a poem. Poems are always read twice, with McLaine saying 'I will read the poem again' after the first reading or the initial response. The frequent initial response of, 'Well, I couldn't make head or tail of that!' is usually followed by a statement that is remarkably, intuitively in touch with the themes of the poem after the second reading. It is in second reading of the poem, when the alchemy of poetry is brought in to the session, that the full sense of the group members listening, taking it in and really being present to the experience is felt. The 'here-and-now' focus is a vital component of the programme at Prague House. Moments of openness and receptivity bring shifts in learning and seeing, and changes in thinking. It is in these moments that the sense of shared experience contributes to a sense of wellbeing.

One poem used in a group session was by Denise Levertov, with the poet comparing the way in which a mountain veiled by cloud becomes invisible to her with the way in which the same mountain disappears for her when she forgets to pay attention to it. The theme struck a familiar chord with participants. After a lively discussion, there was a pause. Two participants, missing their previous night's sleep, sat nodding off. This fact was gently acknowledged. Moments later, postures were alert and the invitation offered to notice, 'What is present here just now?'. 'It is attention!', someone said. Glances and big smiles were exchanged in friendly interactions, the sharing of poetry having brought its magic again.

Reading groups within an informal group learning context

Paulo Freire's pedagogic theory, which he developed in Brazil in the context of adult literacy education, grew out of his passion for social change and what he saw as a need for a kind of education in hope, challenging participants to empower themselves (Leonard and McLaren, 1993). Freire's pedagogic theory is founded on an understanding of 'knowing' as a social activity, inviting group members to participate in an activity of reshaping their understanding of reality in group learning settings. In this sense, 'knowing' means to take on a co-investigator or active co-creator role, encouraging creativity and stimulating true reflection (Eagleton, 2003). This understanding of 'knowing' is an essential part of the Prague House reading group, where the group members' experience includes a self-reflective dimension, with each person engaged in examining their own experience. Iser, (1974, 294) emphasizes that actively involving readers in responding to what they have read in relation to their own experiences 'brings to the fore an element of our being of which we are not directly conscious . . . and so [we] discover what had previously seemed to elude our consciousness.'

Walter, in his early 80s, began to write poetry and said he couldn't live without it. He would be waiting in the room each week and would read aloud to McLaine his weekly writings as she set up the room. Each week Walter and

McLaine would share a few minutes together before the rest of the group gathered. He never wrote or spoke of his own experiences, and said little in the group. When one day he told his own hard story in response to the one being read in one of the sessions, our hearts were touched. After this, Walter said he had 'moved on' from something he had been 'stuck with' about his father.

Mikhail Bakhtin (1981) in his writings awakens us to the effectiveness of dialogue. We use the faculty of language to listen, and then use it to find our own voice and speak what is true for us. Using a dialogical method of facilitation means being both a speaker and listener, as well as inviting participants themselves to be listeners and speakers. For the Prague House marginalized group, whose stories are not typically heard in society, finding the voice to speak what is true for them is an essential element in developing the possibility of group discussion.

Contact with reality seems to be nourished in the reading group for Paul, who suffers from schizophrenia and whose ideas tend to be fixed and judgemental. Paul has said on a number of occasions, particularly with classic stories such as by Dickens, in response to the fictitious plot, 'But that's not real, is it? It's not real'. Paul attends faithfully, listens deeply and says little. The reflective listening to the back-and-forth of the discussion has allowed him to test the ground of his convictions, as Bakhtin maintains, '(w)e author ourselves in conversations with others' (Anderson, 2012, 571).

Social isolation

Social isolation has a major effect on health and wellbeing. Recent studies reveal loneliness is more hazardous to your health than obesity and smoking; it increases the risk of dementia and depression; reduces cancer survival rates; and raises the risk of an early death by as much as 50% (Mercola, 2017). Chronic social isolation is a characteristic of the Prague House residents due to mental health issues, and to the stigma and marginalization they have experienced as a result.

The Prague House reading group favours a model which starts from the life experience and knowledge that group members bring with them to the group (Shor and Freire, 1987). There is a compulsion to share an experience: something that they are giving of themselves that allows others to be part of that journey with them. As well as listening to the texts being read, they also listen to each other. There is a willingness to give time and attention to others. Sharing in this way 'can make visible and 'felt' that which is invisible and 'unfeelable' . . . and lets us stand in the condition of another' (Oliver, 1994,

108).The reading group addresses social isolation through the sense of connection felt in shared participation and shared experience. There is, through reading and listening, both an inner and outer companionship with the words, the images and then with others.

Maurice's contributions in the reading group revealed that he had not lost his ability to use language as was feared, and his articulate and insightful contributions remained a feature of the sessions. However, he was increasingly frail, leading him to isolate himself in his room. The reading group was a programme that encouraged him to leave his bed. When his frailty meant he would need to move to a high-care facility, he came to a final bibliotherapy session, where a story was chosen to allow participants to share warmly with him their appreciation of his contributions and the care and esteem in which they held him.

Meeting the responses of the Prague House reading group

The Prague House group share the 'experience' of reading together rather than sharing the reading. In the Prague House group, changes to the shared reading format occurred to meet the responses of this particular group. A decision was made by the group for the whole story to be read by the facilitator without interruption. What they enjoyed foremost was the melody in a beautiful flowing piece of literature when read aloud. Herman (2006) describes this as the music of speech, similarly aligning the rise and fall of spoken pitch to the pitch in singing or playing an instrument. Oliver (1994, 42) claims that 'rhythm is one of the most powerful of pleasures, and when we feel a pleasurable rhythm we hope it will continue. When it does . . . we are in a kind of body-heaven.' The group members possibly felt this 'body-heaven' as they did not like the reading of stories to stop and start for discussion or to swap readers. What they liked was taking part in the discussion that followed the reading aloud of the text. The narratives and poetry delivered in the reading group provide the vehicle to create a shared moment. The carefully selected texts each week offer the central theme and focus for group discussion. Over time, texts can be chosen that individual group members can relate to, which can help them to reflect on aspects of their lives, offering the group members an opportunity to get to know each other in a more intimate way and for deeper relationships to form.

Group members do, however, choose to share the reading of the poems. After listening to the poem, they individually read the lines of the poem that they have felt drawn too. Paul responds to the poems by reading with depth of feeling the lines that he has chosen. Sometimes this will be the whole poem. We could not have known of Paul's depth of feeling without this programme, and perhaps he would not either. Others also read the lines of the poem they have chosen, while the listeners dwell appreciatively in the moment of present experience: the freshness and surprise of responses, words and the experience of the particular poem are savoured, tasted, turned in the mouth. Using literature in this way involves the notion of the 'savouring of beauty' (Seligman et al. 2009, 306) which can be found in the encounter with beautiful words.

Prague House supports their diverse resident group to live life to the fullest potential. The shared and focused energy of participants in the bibliotherapy sessions is readily apparent to staff and residents who pass by and can see a small dog and a group of people listening and talking with intent. There is a feeling of real calm and uplift that had been created by every single member of the group. Within this group, there is a great sense of connection with people on a deeper level than would occur normally.

The established Prague House reading group is now sustained by Mackenzie and a Prague House volunteer. The Prague House reading group led to the establishment of a new reading group, facilitated by McLaine, in another St Vincent's facility within the criminal justice area. This group takes place within a secure environment and group members are dealing with a range of mental illnesses. This group, set up in 2013, is again demonstrating its ability to complement ongoing formal mental health treatment through offering a different perspective to the more traditional problem-solving forms of therapy. Again, the reading group shows signs of participants improving in the areas of mental health, including a shift in self-awareness, a reduction in social isolation and a change in social dimensions, through supporting, creating and maintaining supportive relationships.

References

Anderson, H. (2012) Peggy Penn in Memoriam: 1931–2012, *Journal of Family and Marital Therapy*, **38** (4), 571–2.

Bakhtin, M. (1981) The Dialogic Imagination. In Holquist, M. (ed. and trans.) and Emerson, C. (trans.), *Four Essays*, University of Texas Press.

Davis, N. (2016) Dogs Understand Both Words and Intonation of Human Speech, *The Guardian*, (30 August), www.theguardian.com/science/2016/aug/30/dogs-understand-both-words-and-intonation-of-human-speech.

Eagleton, T. (2003) *After Theory*, Allen Lane/Penguin.

Freeman-Greene, S. (2011) Between the Lines, *The Age*, (14 March), www.theage.com.au/national/between-the-lines-20110313-1bssj.html#ixzz2gZ8dtnJD.

Herman, D. (2006) Dialogue in Discourse Context: scenes of talk in fictional narrative, *Narrative Inquiry*, **16** (1), 75–88.

Hughes, R. and Szczepek Reed, B. (2017) *Teaching and Researching Speaking; applied linguistics in action*, 3rd edn, Routledge.

Iser, W. (1974) *The Implied Reader: patterns of communication in prose fiction from Bunyan to Beckett*, Johns Hopkins University Press.

Jeannin, S., Gilbert, C., Amy, M. and Leboucher, G. (2017) Pet-directed Speech Draws Adult Dogs' Attention More Efficiently than Adult-directed Speech', *Scientific Reports*, **7** (4980), 1–8.

Leonard, P. and McLaren, P. (eds) (1993) *Paulo Freire: a critical encounter*, Routledge.

Mercola, J. (2017) Loneliness More Hazardous to your Health than Obesity or Smoking, *Mercola*, 24 August, https://articles.mercola.com/sites/articles/archive/2017/08/24/loneliness-hazardous-than-obesity-smoking.aspx?utm_source=dnl&utm_ medium= email&utm_content=art1&utm_campaign=20170824Z3&et_cid=DM155511&et_ rid=26072291.

Mitchell, R. L .C. and Ross, E. D. (2013) Attitudinal Prosody: what we know and directions for future study, *Neuroscience and Behavioural Reviews*, **37**, 471–9.

Oliver, M. (1994) *A Poetry Handbook: a prose guide to understanding and writing poetry*, Houghton Mifflin Harcourt.

Radcliffe, V. F. and Reby, D. (2014) Orienting Asymmetries in Dogs' Responses to Different Communicatory Components of Human Speech, *Current Biology*, **24**, 2908–12.

Seligman, M. E. P., Randal, M. E., Gillham, J., Reivich, K. and Linkins, M. (2009) Positive Education: positive psychology and classroom intervention, *Oxford Review of Education*, **58** (3), 293–311.

Shor, I. and Freire, P. (1987) *A Pedagogy for Liberation*, Bergin & Garvey.

Skidmore, D. and Murakami, K. (2016) Dialogic Pedagogy: an introduction. In Skidmore, D. and Murakami, K. (eds) *Dialogic Pedagogy: the importance of dialogue in teaching and learning*, , Multilingual Matters.

Winnicott, D. W. (2005) *Playing and Reality*, Routledge.

8

Developing a reading group service for an older adult functional psychiatric in-patient ward

David Chamberlain

Background

Bibliotherapy is the therapeutic use of reading to help mental or psychological disorders. There are various methods of delivering bibliotherapy. Firstly, there is the model of clinicians prescribing self-help books, such as those recommended by the National Institute for Health and Care Excellence (NICE) for generalized anxiety (National Institute for Health and Care Excellence, 2011a), common mental health disorders (National Institute for Health and Care Excellence, 2011b) and by the Scottish Intercollegiate Guidelines Network for the non-pharmaceutical treatment of depression (Scottish Intercollegiate Guidelines Network, 2010). Then there is the setting up of themed reading groups (e.g. Kirklees Council, 2014), generally with a facilitator. Finally, there is self-directed reading as highlighted by Chamberlain and colleagues (Chamberlain, Heaps and Robert, 2007).

There is little research on bibliotherapy set within a psychiatric ward and/or hospital, and even less on bibliotherapy in an older adult functional in-patient ward. McLaughlin and Colburn (2012, 14) describe the mechanics of setting up a story and poetry group on an acute mental health ward and highlight the 'transformative power of great literature', seeing the sharing of experience as hugely beneficial. Volpe, Torre, and De Santis (2015) report on a reading group for patients living with psychosis, describing the group as a valid rehabilitation tool. In addition, The Reader has published research (Davies, Billington and Carroll, 2012; The Reader, 2014) on their work for dementia patients in care homes and on a hospital ward, noting 'marked improvements in agitation levels, mood levels and concentration levels for participants, as well as improved social interaction' (The Reader, 2014, 3).

Delivering bibliotherapy

Following an overview of the context to this intervention, the following section discusses the practicalities of introducing bibliotherapy in an older adult psychiatric in-patient ward, in particular, partnership working, group structure and selecting texts.

Context

The library service described in this case study is hosted by an acute trust of medium size (5000 staff across three hospital sites) that also has service level agreements with a health and community trust which includes mental health (4000 staff across three community hospitals); three care commissioning groups; and an ambulance trust (total 2000 staff and four sites). The county is a rural one with hospitals and health centres located across the county.

There are three staffed libraries at the three main acute hospitals' education centres and one drop-in library. There are eight members of staff (six full-time equivalent) divided into three teams: customer care, service development and resource development, as well as site management. The service development librarian's main role is training and literature searches, but this has been extended to partnership working with universities and public libraries and also clinical librarianship with the wards and health departments. Bibliotherapy has a valid role in working with patients in this context and the library's work in this respect has been recognized as an innovation by Health Education England.

The psychiatric unit consists of two 20-bed mixed wards for older people. One is an organic ward (e.g. patients with dementia) the other a functional ward. The latter is where the first bibliotherapy group took place. People on this ward are generally being treated for depression, anxiety, mood disorders and schizophrenia. Two further groups were run after the success of the first group: the second was on another older adult functional psychiatric ward (six months after the first) and the third back on the original ward a year later.

Partnership working

Partnership work is vital for the library services and very often work is created from chance meetings and corridor encounters. Bibliotherapy was an example of this. The health librarian had already set up a Books on Prescription lending scheme for the psychiatric unit and, in discussion with the ward manager, bibliotherapy was mentioned as a therapeutic intervention. The ward manager wanted to develop a group and decided to work with the occupational therapist (OT) to investigate setting up a reading group for the unit. The librarian led on the project, researched the literature and discussed the idea on an online bibliotherapy discussion forum to find out what had been delivered and take any advice offered. He had previously worked as a qualified psychiatric nurse and was familiar with the environment and ethos of the ward.

Once the outline was agreed, the librarian needed to get support from his line manager. Thus a business plan was submitted outlining the group's objectives, risks, expected outcomes and benefits, cost and Trust and regional drivers. Once given the go-ahead, the librarian met with the ward manager and OT to decide on the group structure.

Motivation and drive coming from the ward manager played a part in the number of patients attending and, to some extent, the level of participation within the group. The ward manager and the OT actively engaged in the process: regularly attending, reading aloud and sharing their thoughts and feelings on the poems read. Throughout, there was a feeling of a flattened hierarchy. With the librarian facilitating the group and leading the open discussions, *all* participants could respond to the poems rather than being divided into staff and patients. On the second ward, however, staff were not so motivated to be involved and did not actively engage with the process. The contrast with the first group was pronounced. The ward manager did not lead this group and staff involvement was *ad hoc* depending on nurse activity and rota.

Group structure

Ten one-hour sessions were run weekly with ten different themes. A room was set aside and prepared beforehand for each session. At the beginning, group members introduced themselves by name only and the structure and confidentiality were explained. As with many such groups, ground rules were set at the start of the group, including assuring people they did not need to share any information they did not feel comfortable sharing. It was also agreed with group members that anything discussed during the session would be treated in confidence by other patients in the group. The librarian facilitated the group and was supported by the two therapists. All had previous experience of facilitating groups and working with mental health in-patients. Group numbers ranged from five to 11 patients, and two to three staff.

Selecting texts

The themes initially chosen were: seaside/water, childhood, war, time, favourite poets, nature, love, favourite quotes, holidays and fairy tales. Five or six poems were selected by the librarian on each theme using recommendations from discussion forums and internet sites (e.g. Poetry Foundation, Poetry Soup and Poem Hunter).[1] Copies of the poems were made beforehand and a sheet of pictures relating to the poems was laminated for participates to read from and look at.

Poems were selected as a medium because short stories were considered too long for one session and too singularly focused for the group. As the group was anticipated to be open, as people were discharged and admitted, a book would mean people would not be able to follow the story when they joined the group at different stages and might feel excluded. Short poems allowed people to fully concentrate and follow and contribute to discussions.

Initially staff would read a poem and open the group to discussion using the following structure:

- What was that poem about? What is happening in the text in terms of themes, descriptions, language, etc.
- Did you like it? What may be happening within themselves as individuals in terms of reflection about personal experiences, feelings and thoughts.
- Which poem did you like the best? Contrast and comparison with other poems in the theme.

By simplifying the questions it allowed participants to give their views of what a poem might be about and whether they liked it, with no emphasis on whether their response was right or wrong.

Once the initial format and structure was decided it was easy to adapt when the group was re-run on a different ward and a year later. The themes were changed with fairy tales, favourite quotes and holidays taken out and old age, seasons and Christmas added. The fairy tales were too long to read in one session and elicited little discussion, whilst the quotes were too brief. Old age was added because the nursing team thought this would allow therapeutic discussion; holidays was merged into seasons; and Christmas added to coincide with the time of the year. War poems were also read to coincide with British Remembrance Day. The librarian tried to select archetypical themes which all could relate to.

Evaluating the initiative

The librarian was keen to evaluate the effects of the group. The initial plan for the first group was to hand out simple evaluation forms at the end of each session and for staff to keep reflective diaries. The evaluation form asked, 'What [poem] did you like the best?' 'Can you say why?' 'Did you enjoy the session?' and 'Any other comments?'

The librarian anticipated quite a formal group, with staff briefing and debriefing after each session, where there would be time available to hand out forms. However, this did not happen, as the ward was very busy with patients having individual visits, home visits and meetings, as well as the group finishing close to lunchtime. Thus, after the group, the therapists would leave promptly and the evaluation forms were left on the side for the patients to fill in if they wanted. Only the librarian kept an ongoing diary with the therapists reflecting on the entire experience after the group had ended.

With the final group, however, the librarian decided to set up a more formal approach to data collection using interpretative phenomenological analysis (IPA) (Smith, Flowers and Larkin, 2009). This approach is concerned with trying to understand how participants themselves make sense of their lived experiences. Therefore, it is centrally concerned with the meanings which those experiences hold for the participants. Structured interviews were proposed as a means to collect the necessary qualitative data to explore whether the group was beneficial as a reading group, as opposed to being just a group, and more specifically whether reading aloud made a difference. COREQ (COnsolidated criteria for REporting Qualitative research)[2] was used as a checklist to guide the research.

The nursing staff were responsible for recruiting research participants on the ward and arranging interviews. The difficulty of gaining consent from this client group has been well documented (Clegg et al., 2015) and from the possible 15 participants, four gave consent. Interviews were set up with the in-house psychologist, with two interviews taking place by phone after discharge. The psychologist used the following questions:

- How would you describe yourself as a person?
- Has coming to the reading group made a difference in how you see yourself?
- How did being in a (reading) group make you feel?
- Did reading aloud make a difference to how you felt?
- Was there any particular poem you liked (identified with)?
- Did any poem change how you felt about yourself?

- What was your overall experience of the reading group?

Following the interviews, the ward manager and librarian produced transcripts and then identified themes.

Therapeutic benefits

The librarian analysed the questionnaires and interviews to explore patient experience. The experience of the therapists was provided through their reflections.

Patient experience

From the data provided through the evaluation forms, the experience of the group seemed to be one of empathy and exploration. Participants reflected on their experiences of reading and responding to literature and sharing experiences. Some said they had been motivated to read as a result:

> Inspired to read poetry

> Re-kindled my passion for reading

Others described the ways in which they, or other members of the group, had responded to the experience in ways they did not initially expect to:

> I liked to dissect the poetry and find the meaning – never done that before.

The sharing of responses to the literature was another outcome of the group. Again, this was something that was unexpected for some participants:

> Did her the world of good – normally she doesn't say anything, she opened right up after the war poems in the evening and had us all enthralled for two hours.

> You opened up someone who normally doesn't open up.

The themes identified from the interview transcripts included mutual understanding and shared experience; reminiscence and memories; and enjoyment and empowerment. In general, participants felt empowered through mutual sharing and empathy:

I liked . . . hearing other people's contributions and helps us get to know each other.

I feel like I belong, we are equal to each other. We have all had problems and we are all trying to beat them.

Reading aloud also made a difference and increased participants' confidence and created a sense of self-identity:

It made me feel very important.

Gave me a bit of confidence . . . having thoughts about not being able to do it but thinking to myself, 'I am going to do it; I'm not going to just sit there and be stupid.'

This also helped to make participants feel part of the group; reading was not simply an individual experience:

Allows everyone to contribute as everyone read a verse each . . . people read it their way, (intonation, rhythm, accent, dramatically) . . . you can make it your own.

Felt more involved by reading poetry out loud.

Felt part of what was going on.

For, participants, seeing each other getting well was uplifting and through the group they were able to give support to each other:

Nice listening to other people's thoughts as they had different ideas about the poems . . . people listening to you . . . taking your views seriously even when you are unwell, rather than dismissing you as some sort of idiot.

I was surprised how many people went along . . . made me happy to see how many went along and that there was more people that liked poetry than I realised . . . could see the change in different patients . . . making a big effort to get their lives on an even keel. The group was a good thing not just for me but for others too.

In addition to these benefits the therapists could use particular themes, such as old age, to discuss feelings and emotions in a safe and supportive environment.

The following are reflections written by the key staff members involved: the ward manager, OT and librarian.

Ward manager's reflection

'The ward already offered a number of therapeutic interventions based on relaxation, creative art and social group activities, whilst also supporting interactions relating to daily life and recovery. But there was little on the use of words – words in the sense of self-reflection and offering another way to conveying how someone was feeling.

'The group widened our support and experience for patients whilst supporting them towards their recovery. What was most noticeable was the regular patient attendance. After the first two groups, we did not have to ask a patient twice to attend. They were motivated or easily agreeable, which included a number of clinically depressed patients for whom attending any group was an effort. There was one patient who found getting up in the morning difficult and slow, yet wanted to ensure they attended whenever possible, as they loved reading. Sadly, they found it difficult due to eyesight issues, but loved to listen to the poems being read.

'The regular group attendees' interest also lasted way beyond the session. They could be found reading and sitting together, sharing books, discussing what they had read. I have not seen so many patients taking an active interest in reading in quite the same way before. They became more engaged as a group; they were not simply being brought together through their illnesses alone.

'From observations of patients who attended the group, there was a noticeable increase in their confidence and self-esteem. They felt able to share their ideas, thoughts and interpretations through the group's collective reflections on the poems read. As the group itself grew in confidence, so did the individuals. One particular poem by Edgar Allen Poe called *Alone* resonated with two patients: one with chronic schizophrenia and the other severe anxiety. The patient with schizophrenia said that it captured how he had felt all his life: apart from others and not understood, on the outside looking in. The person with severe anxiety felt that they were not heard and was frustrated by their inability to communicate effectively because they were so anxious. They needed to feel that people understood how they were feeling and the group helped with this.

'One of the most interesting things about the group was that you did not feel like a staff member. Everyone was in the group; everyone took part; and everyone offered their ideas and thoughts as equals. Having an outside facilitator enabled the clinicians to be immersed in the group as participants. This in itself, I feel, changed how we viewed the patients in the group and possibly how the patients viewed us.'

Occupational therapist's reflection

'For those interested in poetry, the group provided an opportunity to participate in a social activity based upon an area of interest. All those who attended the sessions reported finding the group to be an enjoyable social group. Many of the poems led this older adult patient group to reminisce about their life experiences and reflect on both the trials and triumphs of their life to date. In this way, the poems promoted social interaction and participation. A number of patients drew upon parts of poems, making connections between metaphors and imagery depicted in poems to articulate their experience of a range of mental health conditions. These disclosures elicited empathy and support from other group participants in a way that I have rarely observed in other social activity groups, and appeared to be cathartic for patients. This social support appeared to have a carry-over effect outside of the group, with some of the patients joining together in the evening reporting that they had re-read some of the poems from the group. Many patients took copies of the poems at the end of the session stating they would like to read the poems again, providing additional opportunities for engagement in a meaningful occupation.

'In addition to the poetry group providing opportunities for patients to participate in an enjoyable, therapeutic social activity group, it also provided additional assessment opportunities in relation to a range of skills and abilities. Some patients were observed to independently incorporate the group within their weekly routine and to plan their morning routine effectively to ensure they were ready to attend the start of the sessions. In addition, some patients were observed to relax and become less agitated as they focused on listening to the poems. Although no patient was expected to read aloud, almost every patient volunteered to read part of, if not a whole, poem over the course of the group. Observation of patients reading aloud, reading along and turning pages and keeping up with the reader or taking turns to read parts of the poem provided opportunities to assess vision, hearing and concentration. Observation of group discussion provided opportunities to observe patients' communication skills.'

Health librarian's reflection

'The therapeutic group supported the library's strategic drivers to develop partnerships and support patient care. It clearly re-kindled people's love of reading and it was noticeable on the ward that more people were reading books. The more traditional library services were also used, such as literature searches, article requests and training, as the librarian was able to promote services with the ward manager and to staff directly. Public library services were also promoted, with patients and staff becoming aware of the groups available at public libraries, such as 'knit and natter', reading groups and social coffees.'

Conclusion

The setting up and running of a reading group for an older adult functional in-patient ward has been immensely rewarding and enjoyable. For patients, the group was a positive experience; the sharing of poems and the reading aloud acted as a therapeutic trigger for the participants to engage and respect themselves and each other, which seemed to help them on the path of recovery.

Bibliotherapy has since been introduced to other wards and there is a plan to deliver regular yearly reading groups. In addition, through contact with the pastor service, the library staff have spoken to the chaplain and volunteers who have now set up a service reading to patients on the general wards. This has also been recognized as an innovation by Health Education England (2017). In addition, there is potential to use bibliotherapy further as a therapeutic tool, with the themes being tailored for the group and/or individual and with staff using the group as a part of their nursing process for patients.

Notes

1 www.poetryfoundation.org, www.poetrysoup.com, www.poemhunter.com.
2 www.elsevier.com/__data/promis_misc/ISSM_COREQ_Checklist.pdf.

References

Chamberlain, D., Heaps, D. and Robert, I. (2007) Bibliotherapy and Information Prescriptions: a summary of the published evidence-base and recommendations from past and ongoing Books on Prescription projects, *Journal of Psychiatric and Mental Health Nursing*, **15** (1), 24–36.

Clegg, A., Relton, C., Young, J. and Witham, M. (2015) Improving recruitment of older people to clinical trials: use of the cohort multiple randomised controlled trial design, *Age and Ageing*, **44**, 547-550.

Davis, P., Billington, J. and Carroll, J. (2012) A Literature-Based Intervention for Older People Living with Dementia, www.liverpool.ac.uk/media/livacuk/instituteofpsychology/researchgroups/A,Literature-Based,Intervention,for,Older,People,Living,with,Dementia.pdf.

Health Education England (2017) Setting Up and Facilitating a Reading Group on an Elderly Functional Psychiatric Ward, www.libraryservices.nhs.uk/document_uploads/LQAF/Innovation_Results_2017_46d0d.pdf.

Kirklees Council (2014) *Well into Reading*, www.cilip.org.uk/blog/does-bibliotherapy-work.

McLaughlin, S. and Colburn, S. (2012) A Reading Group in Acute Mental Health Care, *Nursing Times*, **108** (44), 14–15.

National Institute for Health and Care Excellence (2011a) *NICE Guidance CG113. Generalised Anxiety Disorder and Panic Disorder (with or without Agoraphobia) in Adults: management in primary, secondary and community care*, www.nice.org.uk/guidance/cg113.

National Institute for Health and Care Excellence (2011b) *NICE Guidance CG123. Common Mental Health Disorders: identification and pathways to care*, www.nice.org.uk/guidance/cg123.

The Reader (2014) *Read to Care: an investigation into quality of life benefits of shared reading groups for people living with dementia*, www.thereader.org.uk/wp-content/uploads/2017/06/Read-to-Care.pdf.

Scottish Intercollegiate Guidelines Network (2010) *Non-pharmaceutical Management of Depression in Adults: a national clinical guideline*, www.sign.ac.uk/assets/sign114.pdf.

Smith, J. S., Flowers, P. and Larkin, M. (2009) *Interpretative Phenomenological Analysis*, Sage.

Volpe, U., Torre, F. and De Santis, V., (2015) Reading Group Rehabilitation for Patients with Psychosis: a randomized controlled study, *Clinical Psychology and Psychotherapy*, **22** (1), 15–21.

9

Bibliotherapy in Uruguay: a case study of the Mario Benedetti Library for patients dealing with substance abuse

Cristina Deberti Martins (translated by Sarah McNicol)

Introduction

Bibliotherapy as a practice dates back to ancient times. An exploration of the uses of reading in various areas of health – both physical and mental – confirms this. However, the conceptualization and investigation of bibliotherapy in academic terms is relatively recent and goes hand in hand with the evolution of the various theories of reading in disciplines such as linguistics, pedagogy, philosophy and psychology that have gained importance since the turn of the century.

This chapter offers an overview of the practice of bibliotherapy in Montevideo, Uruguay, and, more specifically, bibliotherapy within a context of social vulnerability. Being a relatively new discipline in this country, information about bibliotherapy interventions can be scarce or difficult to access. Therefore, the chapter focuses on the specific theory and practice of bibliotherapy in a state health centre, dedicated to the treatment of the problematic consumption of drugs: Portal Amarillo. Bibliotherapy has been developed in Portal Amarillo's library since 2006, and since 2012 training courses have been offered to disseminate the method and encourage its use in other state institutions. The chapter starts with an overview of theories of bibliotherapy relevant to this context before examining the work of Portal Amarillo in more detail.

Theories of bibliotherapy

In 1949, Caroline Shrodes, a student in the USA, defended her doctoral thesis 'Bibliotherapy: a theoretical and clinical-experimental study', laying the theoretical basis of the technique. Shrodes (1960) conceives bibliotherapy as a 'dynamic process of interaction between the reader's personality and the imaginative literature, which can attract his [or her] own emotions and release them to his [or her] conscious and productive use.' For Shrodes, fictional literature is seen as the most appropriate means to achieve internal change. During the 1950s, the technique she described began to spread and many definitions were developed as well as a variety of uses and theoretical frameworks, including bibliotherapy as a discipline, as art, as a technique and as a tool.

The Association of Hospital and Institution Libraries in the USA (1971) officially defined bibliotherapy as 'the use of selected reading materials as therapeutic adjuvants in medicine and psychiatry, also guidance in the solution of personal problems through directed reading'. An alternative definition is offered by Caldin (2001), who defines bibliotherapy as 'directed reading and group discussion, which favours interaction between people, leading them to express their feelings: misgivings, anxieties and desires. In this way the subject shares with the group their experiences and values.' This definition therefore emphasizes the freedom of interpretation on the part of readers as the fundamental element of a bibliotherapeutic dialogue.

In all the definitions, there seems to be a consensus, or common denominator, around the basic principles of the technique, although it has multiple variants. While all the definitions agree on the benefits of reading to provide relief, calm anxieties, find solace and offer recreational opportunities, the modes of application differ, as well as the ideological context and the objectives pursued. Variants of bibliotherapy are specific to the theoretical framework on which they are based, and/or the context in which they are applied, that is, the world of the users that they serve.

The two main categories of bibliotherapy are clinical and recreational. These different approaches depend on the users being treated and whether or not they suffer from recognized mental disorders of various kinds. Thus, in certain health institutions, such as hospitals or sanatoriums, clinical bibliotherapy is used to treat people with specific difficulties that require a certain psychological approach. In these cases, it is usual to work in an interdisciplinary team, where the librarian, who has knowledge of reading materials and can suggest suitable texts, works in conjunction with a psychologist or psychiatrist responsible for patient treatments. When bibliotherapy is framed as cognitive behavioural psychology, directed reading is used and certain readings are advised to help solve problems or to promote a better quality of life. Recreational bibliotherapy, on the other hand, is used for purposes of escapism, solace or entertainment. It usually takes place in public libraries, community spaces and reading clubs. The aim is to socialize; to be part of a group; and to enjoy the pleasure of reading through works of literature. It is important to remember that the boundaries between these models of bibliotherapy are not clear-cut. For example, recreational bibliotherapy can have therapeutic effects or even be transformative in certain situations.

Bibliotherapy in Uruguay

In Uruguay, the practice of bibliotherapy has been, and remains, almost invisible. Knowledge of this 'unofficial' practice comes from teaching techniques developed and verbally disseminated amongst clinical colleagues or allied professionals such as educators and social workers. Examples of locations where bibliotherapy can occur include the Institute for Children and Adolescents of Uruguay (INAU), the State Health Services Administration's (ASSE) Persons Deprived of Liberty (PPL) division, as well as night shelters for people in living on the street who depend on the Ministry of Social Development (MIDES). However, despite this level of activity, a literature search does not reveal more than a small sample of bibliotherapy practices. The published record is therefore not an accurate reflection of the level of activity and the dozens more activities being carried out unrecognized.

In 2005, librarians Lourdes Da Silva, Margarita Sian and Graciela Zorrilla presented a project to create a library for children in the public hospital of Rivera (a city in the north of Uruguay); they included the innovation of implementing bibliotherapy. This was one of the first examples of the implementation of bibliotherapy at an official level in the country. Since 2011, there has been a growing interest in bibliotherapy, to the point that are now students of librarianship and psychology who are interested in the technique and have written their degree theses on the subject (e.g. Bentos, 2017) or presented projects to implement bibliotherapy in their work places (e.g. Delgado del Puerto, 2017). Furthermore, a research project on the influence of bibliotherapy on social reintegration processes has also been developed. This was carried out in the community library of a night shelter run by the MIDES. Other current bibliotherapy activities in Uruguay include the following:

1 Library workshop 'Dreams of Freedom': reading cycles and literary exchanges taking place at the Hospital Vilardebó (a state psychiatric hospital) and supported by a University Extension programme (*Una Biblioteca para Armar*).

2 Community library 'Bibliobarrio': this has been operational since 2009 close to Vilardebó Hospital. People with psychiatric illness are encouraged to work in the library (Cardozo, Corbelo and Sasso, n.d.).
3 Urban Cultural Centre (National Department of Culture): aimed at people living on the streets, but open to the entire community. It has operated since 2010. Its objective is to promote inclusion through cultural practices, including reading.
4 Bibliotherapy with children from INAU homes (Charbonnier and Lorenzelli, 2017): this programme, which started in 2016, is for children who have suffered domestic violence, have difficulties in relationship, low self-esteem and anger management issues. Weekly sessions are held with a maximum of ten children per group and co-ordinated by two specialist psychologists. Ages range between 8 and 12 years old.

Other research focuses on self-help groups for people with eating disorders using self-help books on the subject of food, nutrition and being overweight (Barrios, 2016). In a similar vein, but in another context, reading exploration has been carried out in private residential centres for older adults in Montevideo (Garat, 2010). Furthermore, in relation to reading in prisons, an investigation was carried out on political prisoners during the last military dictatorship (1973–85) (Fuster and Langelán, 2013).

A library for the patients of Portal Amarillo

The population of Portal Amarillo consists of patients whose ages range from 15 to 35 years. They come from vulnerable social or cultural contexts, in some cases, extremely perilous. Most have completed primary education, but have not progressed to secondary level (despite education being compulsory and free in Uruguay until the third year of secondary school).

Staff at Portal Amarillo have been developing bibliotherapy techniques for ten years. The type of bibliotherapy we have created, and which is still undergoing further development, is a blend of what we consider a traditional bibliotherapy, emerging from cognitive behavioural psychology, and psychoanalysis.

The Mario Benedetti Library was created in 2009 within the National Centre for Information and Reference on Drugs. The initiative arose as a result of bibliotherapy practices we were already doing in the centre. This gradually led to the creation of a discrete, and more comfortable, space to carry out bibliotherapy interventions.

Why a psychoanalytical approach?

Our approach to bibliotherapy has its roots in psychoanalysis; we feel that this theory offers a deep and comprehensive understanding of the nature of being human. We are guided in our approach by the theory of Donald Winnicott (1998) and his conceptualization of the 'transitional space'. The transitional space refers to the intermediate zone between the inside (psyche) and the outside (environment); it is an indefinable, invisible, subtle zone: the territory of the imagination, of cultural, of play, of reading and of fantasy. It is a space that is necessary to inhabit in order to transition healthily through what in psychoanalysis is denoted as the process of symbolization. Symbolizing is a complex psychic activity that involves relating ideas, representations, images, voices, words and so forth that are essential to tolerate the absence caused by a loss. If there is a symbol, it is because there is an absence. The possibility of symbolizing is of vital importance in the exposition of a loss; putting into words the psychic pain, the anguish, the sorrow, does not eliminate the suffering but makes it tolerable and therefore helps guard against madness.

Reading offers us precisely that potential safeguard through symbols, words, images and dreams. The words offered by the author of a text often help the reader to come close to putting a name to their affliction and thus function as a link in a chain of symbolism that leads them to better understand their conflicts. The anthropologist of reading Michèle Petit expresses it singularly:

> One of the greatest human anguishes is that of chaos, fragments, divided bodies, of losing the feeling of continuity, of unity. One of the factors by which reading is restorative is that it facilitates the feeling of continuity, the story. A story has a beginning, a development and an end; it enables a union to something. And, sometimes, listening to a story, the chaos of the inner world is appeased and by the secret order that emanates from the work, the interior can also be put in order. The same book object – pages re-joined together – gives the image of a united world. (Petit, 2009)

The population we work with belongs to the so-called 'vulnerable populations' with little symbolic capital and scarce vocabulary, hardly sufficient words to describe the concrete actions of their daily lives. Access to cultural assets is not easy, either; the habit of going to the local library is not encouraged and they exclude themselves from a world they consider does not belong to them: the world of writing is a privilege of others. Thus, just as the mother (or one who fulfils the role of child care) creates a space for the baby that enables it to display its creative potential, so the bibliotherapist must create the right environment for the patient to make contact with new elements in order to develop hitherto hidden capabilities.

The psychoanalytical 'frame'

In psychoanalysis, the 'frame' is conceptualized as a perimeter that separates what is allowed from what is not (Bléger, 1967), and these variables must remain constant in order for the treatment process to take place (Deberti, 2011). The frame has at least three highly useful functions.

1 Firstly, as a research tool, in the sense that, since a certain number of variables remain constant, it is possible to make observations and comparisons for later analysis.
2 Secondly, as a measure that protects both the patient and the clinician, since a third party (the law) determines what is enabled and what is prohibited. It separates what is allowed from what is not.
3 Finally, as an emotional bond generator that guarantees the continuity of experience, and in some cases initiates it. The patients with whom we work usually have the experience of living in a hostile world and therefore feel distrust towards others. The continuity and the stability of the space, and the constant attentive and interested presence of the bibliotherapist, generate feelings of confidence in the reader.

It is important to point out that it is a difficult task to maintain the frame of a given activity in health institutions, since daily emergencies can undermine its stability. Sometimes an urgent situation causes the postponement of the bibliotherapy session, or in serious cases its cancellation. This is why we take great care to respect the time and space afforded for bibliotherapy, but with an attitude of flexibility without which it would be impossible to operate.

Bibliotherapy at Portal Amarillo

Bibliotherapy sessions at Portal Amarillo are held weekly in the reading room; they last one hour and have a maximum number of 12 participants. How do we do it? In a natural, spontaneous and novel way, paying special attention to patients who are interacting with the library for the first time.

Most of them have rarely entered a library and have not had daily contact with books – or if they have, it has been in a school context where the experience has not been pleasant, but on the contrary, left them with feelings of frustration or impotence towards written culture. From patient reactions, we have become aware of the fear that can be generated by the book itself as an object. Far from inviting a patient to open it, books can make them distance themselves, excluding themselves from the experience because they feel they will not understand or will not have the patience to read. At the beginning of the session we all sit around a large table on which we have placed some books, general interest magazines, a poetry game and a box of small sheets of paper (just half a page) containing poems or fragments of prose from texts that we consider beautiful. This selection of texts for their beauty helps us to move away from the more usual types of texts that cater to the supposed interests of these readers. Assisted by the discipline of librarianship (an interdisciplinary field par excellence), we take texts from well known, and lesser-known, authors and with a clinical psychoanalytic attitude, we involve ourselves in the session, letting ourselves be immersed in the experience of reading.

Reading is a phenomenon of extreme complexity; it goes beyond simple decoding of inert signs. Reading mobilizes the senses, generates emotions, activates memories and generates thoughts; it stimulates ideas that are joined with previous representations from older readings. It is a safe harbour in moments of crisis, an emotional shelter before the storms of the soul and warm comfort to the harsh experiences of life. From the 1970s, driven by Iser (1989) and others, there was a change in the way of looking at texts and a turn towards the importance of the reader. In this departure from the absolute primacy of the text emerges an active reader who recreates and gives significance and life to the written page. It is with this notion in mind that we approach the task of bibliotherapy, relying on the capacity of patients (even those who rarely read) to approach the text and start to make it their own.

The selection of a text, which is agreed between the patients and the bibliotherapist, is 'random' in a sense. However, before the meeting, the bibliotherapist is informed by staff providing day-to-day care for patients about events that may have affected group dynamics or the mood of the group, for example, admission or discharge of a patient. Taking account of this, we start the session simply, with open questions about how they feel. We keep the information provided by clinical staff in reserve to use as and when it is pertinent. During the initial conversation, we observe what texts patients are taking to browse and, based on that first selection, we propose a reading. The bibliotherapist starts the reading and at the end (not more than 15 minutes) asks an open question about participants' reactions to what they have heard. Sometimes this question is not understood, especially if patients are focused on concrete thinking and responses. In that case, we re-read the passage and even ask the participants if they would like to read it aloud themselves.

Once patients respond, their answers are usually diverse and varied: in general – and this is surprising for those new to co-ordinating a group – the participants relate the text to what is happening to them at that moment, although this may not be the literal or obvious meaning of the text. In this context, it is helpful to reflect on de Certeau's (1996, 286) conception of the book as the construction of the reader: 'The reader invents in the texts something different to what was intended. He/she detaches them from their origin, combines their fragments and creates something unknown in the space which organizes their possibilities to allow a plurality of meaning.'

Poetry never fails!

Sometimes the texts we offer in the first instance do not generate interest, or even the slightest curiosity, on the part of patients. When that happens, we turn to poetry, which for some reason never fails. Perhaps it is because poetry is, above all, a form of sound. A pleasant sound, because as Friot says, 'poetry makes the words sing, so they say more, and in another way'. Musical words accompany us from earliest childhood, from the first lullaby to children's songs that accompany games; they trigger in almost everyone a sense of joy that produces memories and vivid images. Poetry reunites; articulates language and movement; and captures emotions: hence, 'it escapes any attempt at definition' (Friot, 2016).

To read poetry, we place special emphasis on the voice; we try to control it, so that it is smooth and enveloping. High levels of anxiety in the group often result in chatter and movement, making the task more difficult. When this happens, we must counteract the prevailing mood, reading slowly (and the greater the anxiety, the more slowness is required) and pausing. Little by little, the patients calm down and are able to listen and let themselves be inhabited by the text.

The poem abounds with images, fragrances and colours which trigger memories or experiences of the present, and which bring us distant voices, murmurs of rivers, streets and playgrounds. With this in mind, we turn to Laura Devetach's (2010) concept of the internal 'textoteca'. Devetach refers to text, in a broad sense, as a cultural object and as a means of organizing signs that build meaning. Her theory suggests that all readers (even those who do not consider themselves readers) are criss-crossed by internal texts, consisting of voices, lyrics, sayings and verses which have been accumulated throughout their lives, but they are not aware of. The discovery of this 'textoteca' provides an incentive to continue generating texts, sharing them and putting new words to voices from the past. This process allows patients to narrate their lives, linking the past with the present and projecting themselves into the future. The following vignette offers an example of this in practice.

In one session, a patient asked to read a poem he took from the 'box of borrowed words'. It was a poem entitled *Last Song* by Miguel Hernández, the Spanish poet, and the first verse read:

> Painted, not empty:
> my house is painted
> in the colours
> of great passions and misfortunes.

After the reading, the following exchange took place between patients:

Patient A. (17 years old): 'That poem is really good!'

The other patients (nine in total) nod as they continue to draw and write freely.

Bibliotherapist: 'What did this poem suggest to you?'
Patient C (15 years old): 'What do you mean, "What did it suggest to us"? What do you want us to say? I don't understand . . . I liked how it sounded . . .'
Bibliotherapist: 'I mean, what things does it remind you of, or what does it make you feel? . . . Beyond whether you understood it or not . . . maybe there is nothing to understand . . . What do you think?'
Patient A: 'I liked how it sounded too, and it made me remember my grandmother's house . . .'
Bibliotherapist: 'In what way? What was it like your grandmother's house?'
Patient A: 'It was a very neat house and very clean, there was always a smell of delicious food because my grandmother always cooked . . . nobody made custard like her . . . She died a few years ago . . . she was like my mother . . . more than a mother . . . she was always there.'
Patient D (32 years old): 'It made me think that I don't have a house: I live on the street; I sleep in a night hostel . . . at my age it's a failure . . .'

Patient A: 'Noooo, why? There are stages of life, you are going to have your own house yet . . . '

The session continues to develop in relation to houses of the past, houses from childhood where colours and smells returned that had remained hidden for many years. Some like Patient D reported their current situation, where did not have a house because their problem of substance use had led them to lose family ties, work and, in some cases, even their home. Expressing the anguish this situation caused motivated fellow patients to empathize and in turn to relate similar experiences. In an attempt to articulate past, present and future, the bibliotherapist invited patients to imagine their home in the not-too-distant future. In this way, through their imagination, they could contact their conscious or preconscious desires and project and imagine the situation. Let us not forget that patients who suffer from substance abuse live in the present; they feel disconnected from their past and unable to project themselves into a future. Furthermore, the present they live in is very narrow: everyday life revolves around getting the substance, consuming it, suffering its absence and regaining strength to re-consume.

Most of the members of the group remembered the home where they were born, and the various houses where they lived throughout (often complex, difficult and deprived) childhoods, with the pleasure and the joy of bringing to mind something very precious and almost forgotten. According to Bachelard (1982, 28), the birth house is the main element of psychic integration since, 'it is the first universe of daily life, our corner in the world'. He argues that weighty images, such as those of the house, are charged with symbolism; they relate to solidity, giving the illusion of stability in the face of the challenges of adult life. They offer a private refuge and are associated with the past childhood as a shelter from current adversities.

It is highly probable that the 'success' that poetry has in the sessions has something to do with immediacy, with the brevity of the text and with the urgency that coincides with patients' familiar need to satisfy their addiction. Patients' capacity to delay satisfaction is currently weakened. However, although it is important to support the reader's experience of the text, we must simultaneously try to expand that capacity to delay gratification and thus reduce levels of anxiety.

Conclusion

Our experiences suggest that whatever literary genre is shared in the session, the bibliotherapist needs to keep in mind the degree of complexity involved in the task; the diversity of variables in play; and the certainty that the positive effects of the bibliotherapy session are likely to exceed those we consciously realize. Bibliotherapy as we understand it at Portal Amarillo is a gamble, a proactive attitude and a compelling capacity for enthusiasm.

References

Association of Hospital and Institution Libraries (1971) *Biblio-therapy: methods and materials*, Committee on Bibliotherapy (Mildred T. Moody, chair) and Subcommittee on the Troubled Child (Hilda K. Limper, chair), American Library Association.

Bachelard, G. (1982) *Poética de la Ensoñación*, FCE.

Barrios, C. (2016) *Los Grupos de Autoayuda ALCO: visiones críticas en el abordaje terapéutico de la obesidad*, unpublished.

Bentos, C. (2017) La Bibliolterapia como Función Clave en las Bibliotecas para Pacientes con Adicción a las Drogas, unpublished.

Bléger, J. (1967) Psychoanalysis of the Psycho-analytic Frame, *International Journal of Psycho-Analysis*, **48** (4), 511–19.

Caldin, C. (2001) A Leitura como Funcao Terapeutica: biblioterapia, *Encontros Bibli: revista eletrônica de biblioteconomia e ciência da Informação*, **12**, 1–16.

Cardozo, D. Curbelo, T. and Sasso, L. (n.d.) *Centro Cultural y Biblioteca Bibliobarrio*, www.psico.edu.uy/bibliobarrio.pdf.

Charbonnier, A. and Lorenzelli, G. (2017) *Imaginando Junto a Otros*, unpublished.

Deberti, C. (2011) Biblioterapia: propuesta de un encuadre, *Itinerario: revista del Instituto de Psicología Clínica de la Facultad de Psicología de la UdelaR*, www.itinerario.psico.edu.uy/revista%20anterior/Biblioterapiapropuestadeunencuadre.htm.

De Certeau, M. (1996) *Leer: una cacería furtiva*, ITESO.

Delgado del Puerto, V. (2017) *Biblioterapia: una estrategia posible para favorecer los procesos de inclusión social*, unpublished.

Devetach, L. (2010) *La Construcción del Camino Lector*, Comunicarte.

Friot, B. (2016) Nécessaire Poésie, *Guides des Lectures de Lire et Faire Lire*. Imp Flash (unnumbered pages).

Fuster, Y. and Langelan, C. (2013) La Lectura Perforando los Límites de la Cárcel: una mirada sobre las presas políticas en el Uruguay de la dictadura (1973–1985), *Informatio*, **18** (2), 77–102.

Garat, S. (2010) *La Lectura en los Residenciales para Adultos Mayores de la Ciudad de Montevideo*, unpublished.

Iser, W. (1989) *Prospecting: from reader response to literary anthropology*, Johns Hopkins University Press.

Petit, M. (2009) La Lectura Construye a las Personas, *Revista Ñ*, http://edant.revistaenie.clarin.com/notas/2009/06/29/_-01948893.htm.

Shrodes, C. (1960) Bibliotherapy: an application of psychoanalytic theory, *American Imago*, **17**, 311–19.

Rodriguez, S. and Da, L. (2005) *Propuesta de una Biblioteca Infantil Hospitalaria; aporte a la incorporación de la biblioterapia en el Hospital de Rivera*, unpublished.

Winnicott, D. (1998) *Realidad y Juego*, Gedisa. (*Playing and Reality*, 2005, Routledge).

10

Adapting the Books on Prescription model for people living with dementia and their carers

Rosie May Walworth

An introduction to Reading Well Books on Prescription for dementia

Reading Well Books on Prescription for dementia is a book list of quality-assured reading to support people with dementia, and their carers and relatives, through living with dementia. The scheme is part of the wider UK national Reading Well Books on Prescription programme which was developed by the Reading Agency in partnership with the Society of Chief Librarians (SCL) and is delivered through public library services across England. The concept of the programme is simple yet effective: providing book-based support to people living with a range of conditions which is then available for them to borrow free from their local library. Users can either receive a recommendation of a title from a health or social care professional or they can self-refer to the scheme simply by visiting the library and taking one of the books off an open shelf. There are also Reading Well Books on Prescription lists to support adults with common mental health conditions, young people's mental health and wellbeing, and people with long-term physical health conditions and their carers.

The Books on Prescription model was first developed in Wales in 2005 by Professor Neil Frude and was adopted with his support across England in 2013. In 2015, The Reading Agency and SCL then developed the first Books on Prescription list for people with dementia and their carers, with the support of a wide range of partners from the health and social care sectors. Every book on the list has gone through a thorough book selection process with a panel of health experts and people living with dementia. The books provide information and advice; support for living well; advice for relatives and carers; and personal stories. Each of these categories was included for its individual value to users and its unique contribution to the book list as a whole.

Identifying the need

Before starting a new Books on Prescription style intervention, it is essential to identify the need for a scheme and assess whether any potential scheme will address a need in wider society. Taking advice from colleagues in public health can assist with this. At the time of development in 2015, we identified a clear need for people with dementia. Dementia care was identified as a key government policy priority after several influential Department of Health reports recommended dramatic changes in how dementia was viewed and reviewing the adequacy and design of service provision, ranging from early diagnosis and primary care through to acute and residential care (Department of Health, 2013). The then Prime Minister, David Cameron, had also just announced the Prime Minister's challenge on dementia which had a focus on awareness, quality care and research (Department of Health and the Rt Hon David Cameron, 2012). A Books on Prescription scheme for people with dementia supported two of these focuses: providing a clear path to raising awareness for people with dementia as well as providing a service to support care quality improvement.

The thorough process of mapping current policy and provision around dementia had demonstrated that there was a clear need to develop a Books on Prescription scheme for people with dementia and their carers; the next step would be to develop a scheme to effectively address this need.

Developing the scheme

The development of the dementia scheme was modelled on the best-practice approach that had been used to develop the original scheme for adult common mental health conditions. The process was split roughly into the following phases: consultation, partnership development, book selection and design of materials, before preparation for the national launch.

The consultation phase

The consultation phase of each Reading Well Books on Prescription scheme is key to the success of the programme. For the dementia scheme, an external health consultant developed a detailed consultation paper which considered the key areas of need, policy and evidence base that related to the development of the new scheme (The Reading Agency and Society of Chief Librarians, 2013). The consultation paper was circulated to a wide range of relevant professional health bodies and experts to gain consensus on the priorities for the scheme.

The consultation paper also considered recommended aims and outcomes of the new scheme which were developed in response to the need and current policy priorities identified. For example, it was noted in the consultation paper that there are over half a million people caring for people with dementia in England and that one in three people can expect to care for someone with dementia during their lifetime. Therefore, an additional recommended outcome of the scheme was supporting relatives and carers (The Reading Agency and Society of Chief Librarians, 2013).

Partnership development

The development of key partners with expertise in the health and social care sector is hugely important to the development of the Reading Well Books on Prescription programme, and was even more so in the development of the dementia scheme. The Reading Agency and SCL, who facilitated this partnership development, first had to identify organizations and networks with the essential knowledge and expertise required to support the development of the scheme from the consultation phase, through to the book selection, and the design of materials.

Mapping of partners resulted in support from key sector organizations including the Alzheimer's Society, The British Psychological Society, Innovations in Dementia and the Royal College of Psychiatrists. Representatives from these key partners then played an essential part in feeding into the development of the book list, allowing the scheme to benefit from the breadth and depth of knowledge and understanding provided by their wide-ranging knowledge of dementia and dementia care. As a best practice example of partnership working, those with expertise in developing a Books on Prescription list and experts in the field of dementia worked in synergy to produce a list of high-quality relevant titles.

These national partners have also been an essential delivery mechanism on a local level for public libraries, who have worked in partnership with local dementia organizations to effectively promote and deliver the scheme.

Design of materials

Supporting promotional resources, in particular leaflets and posters, provided signposting to the scheme in public settings including libraries, health practices and care homes, as well as digitally for those searching for support online. These supporting resources needed to be useful and accessible for people with dementia to ensure that the Books on Prescription model would work effectively with their specialized needs. Ensuring accessibility of materials for people with dementia on a basic level involves ensuring that design areas such as font and colour are dementia-friendly.

Book selection

In the development of the original Reading Well Books on Prescription scheme for adult common mental health conditions, the strategy for gathering evidence relied heavily on recommendations about the use of guided self-help books or self-help groups contained within the relevant National Institute for Health and Care Excellence (NICE) guidance (National Institute for Health and Care Excellence, 2017). Where there was evidence of ineffective or potentially harmful self-help interventions, these books were not included. Given that the majority of books offering self-help were for identified conditions/problems where NICE guidance was available, this ensured that an identifiable and transparent evidence base was deployed.

When conducting a review of recommended literature for the dementia scheme, it became clear that the majority of titles did specifically identify the form of dementia or neurodegenerative condition, but used dementia as an umbrella term. The similarity of experiences of managing individual dementias or Alzheimer's disease meant that referring to specific clinical conditions or problems was less relevant. Moreover, the majority of titles recommended for dementia tended to be orientated educationally towards increasing information and understanding and offering both practical and emotional advice and support. This contrasted with the titles on the Reading Well Books on Prescription common mental health list, which were all self-help genre and aimed to offer self-administered or guided therapy. It was therefore decided that that it was best to focus on different types of interventions suggestion for people with dementia rather than on specific conditions.

The book selection process to develop the dementia scheme balanced the inclusion of non-fiction, fiction and memoir. The book selection process aimed to provide a range of services for those living with dementia, with each area demanding its own framework for book selection. These services translated into the following categories in the book list:

- information and advice
- support for living well

- advice for relatives and carers
- personal stories.

Information and advice

The policy paper *A National Dementia Strategy: living well with dementia* (Department of Health, 2009) outlined a strategy to ensure significant improvements in dementia services. The strategy identified 17 key objectives, implemented largely at a local level, which aimed to improve services and promote a greater public understanding of the causes and consequences of dementia. The first objective was *improving public and professional awareness and understanding* and a further objective was *good-quality information for those with diagnosed dementia and their carers*. Both objectives led to the important inclusion of an information and advice section of the scheme. The inclusion of information and advice also followed clinical guidelines on dementia: 'increasing knowledge of dementia and gain understanding of the experiences that people with dementia share' (National Institute for Health and Care Excellence, 2006).

The *information and advice* section of the list includes information on normal ageing and memory problems; general information about dementia; and a title suitable to read to, or be read by, children. The general information titles about dementia have been particularly popular, with *Understanding Alzheimer's Disease & Other Dementias* and *Coping with Memory Problems* being in the top five most loaned titles in the 2016/17 evaluation (The Reading Agency and The Society of Chief Librarians, 2017). The information title aimed at children, *Grandma,* has been one of the most borrowed titles on the dementia list. The popularity of this title has demonstrated the benefit of the scheme to parents and young children living with a relative with dementia, and how information provision for children around dementia is an effective addition to the Books on Prescription model.

Support for living well

Living well with dementia was another essential area that was flagged up through policy mapping. Research has stressed the importance of people with dementia remaining as independent and active as possible through involvement with social activities and support groups (Bates, Boote and Beverley, 2005; Brodaty, Green and Koschera, 2003; Cooper et al., 2012). Therefore these titles aim to provide advice and activities for people with dementia and their carers to actively work towards improving quality of life.

For example, *First Steps to Living with Dementia* by Dr Simon Atkins talks about the steps before and after diagnosis; legal and financial support for living with dementia; and active methods of dealing with 'troublesome symptoms'. *Hearing the Person with Dementia: Person-Centred Approaches to Communication for Families and Caregivers*, by Bernie McCarthy, covers methods of verbal and non-verbal communication; techniques for communicating with people who cannot speak or move easily; and strategies for communicating more effectively in specific day-to-day situations. This title addresses the support carers need particularly in the later stages of dementia.

The *Living well with dementia* section also includes activities to share between people with dementia and their families and carers. This includes the title *Chocolate Rain*, which provides ideas for creative approaches to activities within dementia care. This title is unique in the field of living well with dementia. It includes more than 100 successfully tested ideas for a wide range of new activities and is one of the first creative manuals written specifically for caregivers. These resources enable carers to engage in activities with people with dementia that can improve their quality of life and their wellbeing.

Advice for relatives and carers

The challenges of caring for someone with dementia are well researched and the importance of supporting carers both practically and emotionally throughout the dementia journey is emphasized by the Department of Health, NICE and charities including Alzheimer's Society and Carers Trust, and professional bodies. It was clear that aside from people with dementia themselves, informal and formal carers would be one of the main audiences for the dementia scheme.

The *advice for relatives and carers* section covers both practical and emotional support for carers and relatives of people with dementia. *When Someone You Love has Dementia* by Susan Elliot-Wright looks at practicalities and relationships, information on medications and types of therapy, outside help and services and how to access them, and the financial and legal side of caring for someone with dementia. Other titles provide wider support for friends and relatives who are perhaps not the sole carer, *Dementia: support for family and friends* is written specifically for friends and relatives; it explores each stage of the 'journey with dementia' and explains not only how it will affect the person with the condition, but also those around them.

It was important when developing the scheme to also consider particular groups who might struggle to access some of the other titles in the section in terms of accessibility. There are therefore titles that are written to support people with lower reading levels and learning disabilities (*Can I Tell You about Dementia? A guide for family, friends and carers* by Jude Welton) and for the huge number of carers for whom English is a second language (*Seeing beyond Dementia: A handbook for carers with English as a second language* by Rita Salomon).

Personal stories

The inclusion of personal stories was an essential demand of the people with lived experience of dementia who were involved in the book selection process. They recognized the importance to people with a diagnosis of dementia, and their carers, to see their experiences reflected in memoirs and stories on the list. *Still Alice* by Lisa Genova, the story of a university professor who develops early-onset Alzheimer's, which was later turned into a film, was endorsed hugely by those living with dementia. They felt the experiences, thoughts and feelings of the character represented their own and that this was an important reason to include the title on the list.

Books on Prescription had previously only provided non-fiction titles focused on self-help and self-management techniques. The inclusion of fiction and personal stories on the dementia list demonstrated how the Books on Prescription model was adapted to work most effectively for people with dementia. This also demonstrated the importance of engaging people with lived experience of a condition in the development of a Books on Prescription list.

Including fiction and memoir involved having to develop a framework to decide desired outcomes of personal stories included on the list, and therefore a criterion for inclusion and exclusion of titles. It quickly became clear that the main outcome of including personal stories was representing the diverse range of experiences of people living with dementia. Interestingly, the adaptation of the Books on Prescription model to include personal stories in order to support people living with dementia has now widened the footprint of other aspects of the Reading Well Books on Prescription programme.

Delivering the dementia scheme in the public library setting

The Books on Prescription model was a nationally developed initiative. All of the Reading Well Books on Prescription schemes are delivered primarily through local authority public library services, and allow for the schemes to sit at the heart of the community. In adapting the Books on Prescription model for people with dementia and their carers, it was clear that public libraries would continue to be the best space to offer the service.

The SCL Universal Health Offer for Public Libraries expresses the public library contribution to the positive health and wellbeing of local communities (Society of Chief Librarians, 2016). Sitting under this wider offer is the Universal Public Library Dementia Offer. The dementia offer is a national strategy to raise public awareness of dementia and help people with dementia and their carers to understand and live with dementia; access appropriate support; engage in therapeutic activity; and remain independent, active and engaged for as long as possible (The Reading Agency and Society of Chief Librarians, 2013). The commitment demonstrated through the Public Library Dementia Offer to make public libraries a free, safe community space for people with dementia is central to its suitability as a setting for a Books on Prescription scheme for people with dementia and their carers.

Public libraries across England deliver regular events and promotions to support people with dementia in their communities and often have a programme of activity designed to support this. From running dementia cafés to self-help groups for carers, community libraries lead by example on providing dementia-friendly community spaces. An example of this best practice was the programme of events Southwark Heritage and Libraries put together for Dementia Awareness Week 2017 (Southwark Local History Library and Archive, 2017). The library service put on a series of relaxed drop-in activities designed for people living with dementia, their families and carers, and for anyone who wanted to reminisce and share stories about Southwark's past, with everything from dementia awareness training to sessions on the local history of Southwark.

The regular use of the public library setting to support people in the community living with dementia confirms the significance of using the public library space to deliver the Reading Well Books on Prescription scheme for people with dementia. Evidence that shows the library space is comforting, calming and empowering (Brewster, 2014), all of which is inductive to positive experiences for people with dementia.

A case study: the Pictures to Share titles and reminiscence therapy

The second most popular titles on the Reading Well Books on Prescription list are the Pictures to Share collection. Pictures to Share are a social enterprise who develop visual media for people with mid-to-late-stage dementia and a range of other degenerative conditions. The titles were added to the dementia scheme list to support carers and relatives to engage in reminiscence therapy with people with dementia, which has proven benefits both to people with dementia and for those caring for them.

Library services often loan out the Pictures to Share titles to care homes. After borrowing the Pictures to Share titles from the local library in Gosforth, Newcastle upon Tyne, an activities co-ordinator at a nearby care home shared stories of the positive effects the collection had had on the residents. She explained:

> I was searching on my local library website, looking to set up a little library for our residents and also looking at items which may be suitable for people who have dementia when I came across the Pictures to Share collection. The Pictures to Share titles are large hard-backed books, each with a different theme, including sport, the countryside, family life and the seaside. They are filled with beautiful photos, pictures and quotes.
>
> One day, I came across a lady with dementia who sat flicking through one of the titles and chuckling away. We had a guest speaker come in that day, but she was just so enthralled by the book that at one point during the talk she interrupted saying 'Excuse me, can I just ask a question?' We all turned and she said 'Why did the chicken cross the road?' and proceeded to laugh, as did the rest of us. If on other days this same lady appeared unsettled, the books always came to the rescue.
>
> Another lady, who is very happy and always wants to dance, called me over; she was looking at a photo of a boy and his mum smiling and the caption 'Smile and the world smiles with you.' The lady pointed to the caption and then started to sing. It was a beautiful moment and brought a tear to my eye, as well as hers.
>
> I have never seen a book with so few words evoke such emotionally positive reactions. I have had residents open up about their past from seeing photos in the book. If a resident perhaps isn't very vocal or tends to not wish to take part in much, these books are a way to engage with them. I am so happy that I found these books.

User feedback on the scheme

There has been an overwhelmingly positive response to the Reading Well Books on Prescription scheme for dementia. In the 2016/17 annual evaluation of the programme (The Reading Agency and Society of Chief Librarians, 2017):

- 96% of respondents to a user survey found the book helpful (46%) or very helpful (50%)
- 73% of respondents reported that the book had increased their awareness of sources of help
- 63% of respondents reported that the book had helped them to understand more about dementia
- 57% of respondents reported that the book had helped them to care for someone with dementia
- 39% of respondents reported that the book had supported them to cope better with the illness.

These findings were in line with previous years and show that the key aims and outcomes outlined in the development of the scheme were being achieved in practice. The report also demonstrated who was using the scheme and that 73% of users surveyed were relatives or carers of someone who has dementia, confirming the importance of including materials for relatives and carers in the scheme. The majority of respondents were also members of their local library (92%) which validates again the decision to place the Books on Prescription scheme within the public library.

The Reading Agency and the SCL have done a huge amount of positive learning in the development and delivery of a Books on Prescription service for people with dementia and their carers. The Books on Prescription model has adapted effectively to suit this complex population and has been successful in meeting the needs outlined prior to development.

References

Bates, J., Boote, J. and Beverley, C. (2004) Psychosocial Interventions for People with a Milder Dementing Illness: a systematic review, *Journal of Advanced Nursing*, **45**, 644–58.

Brewster, L. (2014) The Public Library as Therapeutic Landscape: a qualitative case study, *Health and Place*, **26**, 94–9.

Brodaty, H., Green, A. and Koschera, A. (2003) Meta-analysis of Psychosocial

Interventions for Caregivers of People with Dementia, *Journal of American Geriatrics Society*, **51**, 657–64.

Cooper, C., Mukadam, N., Katona. C., Lyketsos, C. G., Ames, D., Rabins, P., Engedal, K., de Mendonca Lima, C., Blazer, D., Teri, L., Brodaty, H. and Livingston, G. (2012) Systematic Review of the Effectiveness of Non-pharmacological Interventions to Improve Quality of Life of People with Dementia, *International Psychogeriatrics*, **24**, 856–70.

Department of Health (2009) *A National Dementia Strategy: living well with dementia*, www.gov.uk/government/publications/living-well-with-dementia-a-national-dementia-strategy.

Department of Health (2013) *Dementia: a state of the nation report on dementia care and support in England*, www.gov.uk/government/publications/dementia-care-and-support.

Department of Health and the Rt Hon David Cameron (2012) *Prime Minister's Challenge on Dementia*, www.gov.uk/government/news/prime-minister-s-challenge-on-dementia.

National Institute for Health and Care Excellence (2006) *Dementia: supporting people with dementia and their carers in health and social care (CG42)*, www.nice.org.uk/guidance/cg42.

National Institute for Health and Care Excellence (2017) *Improving Health and Social Care through Evidence-based Guidance*, www.nice.org.uk.

Society of Chief Librarians (2016) *Universal Health Offer*, http://goscl.com/universal-offers/health-offer.

Southwark Local History Library and Archive (2017) *Living Memories: a programme of events for Dementia Awareness Week 2017*, www.wise16.co.uk/living-memories-a-programme-of-events-for-dementia-awareness-week-2017.

The Reading Agency and Society of Chief Librarians (2013) *Reading Well Books on Prescription Scheme for People with Dementia and their Families and Carers: consultation paper*, https://readingagency.org.uk/resources/RWBOP%20Dementia%20Consultation%20paper.pdf.

The Reading Agency and Society of Chief Librarians (2017) *Reading Well Books on Prescription: evaluation of year 4 – 2016/17*, https://tra-resources.s3.amazonaws.com/uploads/entries/document/2480/171009_TRA_RWBoP_Y4_Evaluation_-_Final.pdf.

11

Engaging young people in bibliotherapy and reading for wellbeing

Rosie May Walworth

Introduction

As a result of the success of the Reading Well Books on Prescription programme with the development of both the adult mental health and dementia schemes, The Reading Agency and the Society of Chief Librarians (SCL) decided in 2015 to extend the programme to cater for young people. This was the first time a Reading Well Books on Prescription scheme had not focused primarily on an adult audience and the challenge of engaging young people in a reading for wellbeing programme was acknowledged.

The main challenge was presented by the fact that young people tend to engage less with reading-based activity than any other age group. Research shows that 44% of young people aged 16–24 do not read for pleasure (The Reading Agency, 2017) and many young people have negative attitudes to reading, with 28% of young people saying that they only read when they have to (Statista, 2017).

It was clear, however, that there was an evident need for a Books on Prescription-style intervention to support young people's mental health and wellbeing. The increasing challenges around young people's mental health and wellbeing have been well documented in the media in recent years and there are statistics that confirm these assertions. The Mental Health Foundation (2017) note that: 20% of adolescents may experience a mental health problem in any given year; 50% of mental health problems are established by the age of 14; and up to 70% of children and adolescents who experience mental health problems have not had appropriate interventions at a sufficiently early age. Contemporary pressures, such as widespread family breakdown, school exam stress, 24-hour social networking and an increase in bullying, have serious implications for the mental health of young people.

The need for this intervention for young people therefore outweighed the possible challenges that might be faced during development and delivery. This chapter outlines the measures that have been taken both in the development and delivery of the scheme that have ensured its success in engaging young people.

About Reading Well for young people

Reading Well for young people is the third strand of the Reading Well Books on Prescription programme, and is developed in partnership with The Reading Agency, the SCL and the Association for Senior Children's and Education Librarians (ASCEL). The scheme is aimed at 13–18 year-olds to support their mental health and wellbeing through a curated book list of information and advice, endorsed by health experts and young people themselves.

The book list of 35 titles covers the following common mental health conditions in young people: attention deficit hyperactivity disorder (ADHD); anxiety and panic; autism and Asperger syndrome; body image and eating disorders; bullying; confidence and self-esteem; depression; mood swings; obsessive compulsive disorder (OCD); self-harm; and stress. It also features a number of general titles that cover life experiences such as bereavement; divorce and separation; sexuality; sleeping problems; and substance abuse. The books come in a wide range of reading levels and formats, including self-help, fiction, psychoeducation and graphic novels.

Reading Well for young people developed its approach via a consultation which follows National Institute for Health and Care Excellence (NICE) guidelines for common mental health issues and specific mental health issues in children and young people (The Reading Agency, 2015). The books were selected by health professionals following a rigorous and evidence-based approach and the scheme has been co-produced with young people.

The young people's scheme was launched in April 2016, and since its launch, the books on the list have issued over 127,117 times in public libraries alone, with a 152% increase in loans compared to the previous year (The Reading Agency and Society of Chief Librarians, 2017). This data does not include the huge number of young people accessing the books through school and college libraries. The scheme has also had an incredibly positive reception from young people. Early findings show that 96% of young people surveyed report that the book had provided support in dealing with difficult feelings and experiences; 87% reporting that it had provided advice for coping with pressures associated with mental health and wellbeing; 77% reporting that it had provided useful information and advice; and 59% reporting that the book had helped to boost their confidence (The Reading Agency and Society of Chief Librarians, 2017).

Gathering youth insight

As a first step in the development of a Reading Well Books on Prescription scheme for young people, The Reading Agency commissioned co-creation specialists Latimer to produce a youth insights report on perceptions of mental health; reading for education and pleasure; existing mental health campaigns; and the perceptions of the existing Reading Well Books on Prescription programme (Latimer Group, 2015). They delivered two two-hour insight sessions with participants aged 13–18 from London.

A huge amount of learning came out of the report and young people were positive both about reading and about public libraries. The key messages from the report were as follows: the importance of schools in the success of the scheme; the clear market for the scheme; the importance of peer recommendations; and the position of the scheme as a resolution to self-diagnosis.

Throughout the report, young people cited school as a constant consideration. When discussing offline habits, school was constantly referred to as a space of emotional and physical engagement. It was also noted, when discussing library engagement, that school libraries needed to be a key delivery partner. Young people were happy to use their local public library as a study space and to find new material to read, but they regularly referred to the importance of the school library, too. This was particularly the case amongst the younger ages, who had slightly less social freedom to explore amenities outside school. As a result of this, Reading Well for young people is marketed directly to schools and educational professionals, making sure that all the materials are still signposting young people to their public library.

The young people in the insight sessions applauded the existing Reading Well programmes and reacted positively towards the concept and the materials. The report cited the real market for a Books on Prescription scheme for young people, noting that young people are interested in boosting their mental health and wellbeing, but often feel at a loss as to how to take control of their own mental health. This, alongside the report noting that young people saw the scheme as a resolution to the dangers of self-diagnosis, gave acknowledgement to the fact that a young people's list would be positively received by its intended audience.

Peer recommendation was also cited as key, with one young person saying 'If I have a tip from someone else, I'll give it a chance'. This peer recommendation was one of the main motives for going on to co-produce the book list with young people. It was clear that if young people could see the books had been chosen and read by their peers, they would be more likely to pick them up and read them.

Co-producing the book list

The clear benefit of engaging with young people themselves to develop the scheme led to the decision to invite external organizations to tender for a co-production strand of the Reading Well for young people development. This process resulted in the commissioning of national youth mental health charity, YoungMinds, to deliver an extensive co-production process to run alongside the book selection panel made up of experts from professional health bodies and charities.

This process was split into two phases: book selection and design of materials; and promotions strategy. YoungMinds recruited six young advisors who led the co-production work as experts by experience. These young advisors then worked in partnership with staff from YoungMinds to develop and deliver workshops for young people across the country.

There was much learning in the early stages of the co-production process. The young advisors highlighted key issues for themselves and their peers. In an initial discussion about the scheme, prior to the workshops, the young advisors noted the following:

1 For young people to take out any of the titles from a library it is important for them to know they are there in the first place – promotion is essential.
2 There was agreement that books can play an important role in improving mental health.
3 The scheme could be particularly useful for young men who do not want to admit they need help.
4 The possible risk of books becoming an emotional or psychological trigger, associated with bad memories for anyone reading them, and how this could be avoided.
5 The importance of inclusion of books on the impact of mental health issues as well as overtly about mental health.

The young advisors then devised and delivered workshops to shortlist titles from a longlist provided by The Reading Agency. This used shortlisting criteria which were developed by young advisors and The Reading Agency and simplified into a list. The shortlisted titles needed to:

- be suitable for 13–18-year -olds
- have a young-people-friendly design
- contain reliable information, advice or support
- be of sufficient depth and detail of topic
- be accessible for diverse readers
- be an appropriate length
- contain interesting graphics or images
- use positive terminology
- have clarity about possible 'triggers'
- not be stigmatizing
- provide practical advice
- provide a message of hope
- be real to the reader.

The young people then met to discuss the titles and whether they fulfilled these criteria. They used activities and interactive discussions around the fiction and non-fiction titles respectively. With fiction in particular, books were popular when they seemed relatable. Conversations often centred around the importance of representing different sexualities, race and religion. For non-fiction, participants discussed how important it was for the books to be well written and to be attractive to their age group. In particular, titles also needed to not be too long and to use simple language.

Throughout the co-production workshops, it became apparent that the current Reading Well Books on Prescription title of the scheme was liked by some of the young people, but heavily rejected by others. This led to a discussion over possibly re-imagining the name of the scheme and it was renamed Reading Well for young people. The continued use of 'Reading Well' ensured brand recognition for the programme. The young people also added in the tagline 'find Shelf Help in your local library' which is used on the leaflet and posters, and has resulted in the scheme often being referred to informally as Shelf Help.

A final report from the young people highlighted their recommendations and commendations. They endorsed the importance of books being available free and for health and education professionals to be able to recommend the books to young people they are working with. The titles were seen as accessible and appealing to the diverse range of preferences that young people have. The young people also flagged up that the marketing of the scheme and the distribution of the books needed to consider the potential of books acting as emotional or psychological triggers for readers feeling emotionally unwell and the importance of the leaflets and website information signposting to other sources of information and support.

Using activity to engage young people with the scheme

After the national launch of the Reading Well for young people scheme in April 2016, The Reading Agency and SCL were keen to ensure as many young people as possible had the opportunity to engage with the list. The Reading Agency provided public libraries with a range of ideas and resources to promote the scheme and heavily encourage library services to work with local partners (such as schools and youth organizations), as well as with young people themselves, to promote the scheme to young people throughout their community and make them aware of the resource available to them. This approach has been regularly used through libraries in England. For example, young people from Watford organized a launch event for the young people's scheme at their local library, inviting local Child and Adolescent Mental Health Services (CAMHS) and youth organizations Youth Connexions and 0–25 Together to attend a launch event. Young people in Suffolk libraries even made a short film about the scheme (Suffolk Libraries UK, 2016).

Young people have also been encouraged to develop new and innovative ways of engaging with the scheme. Working closely with The Reading Agency's young people's programme, Reading Hack, young people have been encouraged online and in libraries to develop activities for themselves and their peers around the list, its content and wider discussions around mental health and wellbeing.

The Reading Agency and Lewisham libraries received a small amount of additional funding to work with young people to develop a programme of activity based on the Reading Well for young people list. Staff at Lewisham libraries worked with a group of young people at Somerville Youth Centre in New Cross. Over the course of six weeks, young people read short extracts from the titles on the list and discussed their experiences around the topics of bullying, stress, gender and sexuality (all of which are covered in titles on the book list). The young people developed activities around these topics and used them as stimulus for engaging in discussions around them. They ran a 'stress hack', where the young people wrote down the things that made them feel stressed on stones. They then used the words on the stones as a starting point for writing haikus. This kind of engagement with the list as a first step for creatively engaging with mental health and wellbeing proved to be incredibly positive.

Developing a school-based approach to the scheme

At the start of 2017, The Wellcome Trust commissioned the University of Westminster to conduct an independent qualitative study on the Reading Well for young people scheme which took place in a school environment (University of Westminster, 2017). The evaluation was extremely positive about the scheme itself, but also provided important learning about how the scheme could be used in a mediated environment such as a school. This also allowed an opportunity to respond to the significance placed on the school environment by the young people involved in development.

The evaluation placed multiple copies of the Reading Well for young people list in a school and a local youth counselling service, and young people were left to interact with the books for three months. The engagement with the books was monitored at each site. Young people and key adult stakeholders participated in focus groups and interviews. Qualitative analysis was then used to determine the impact of engaging with the scheme, with 33 participants (15 adults and 18 young people) providing data.

The evaluation identified innovative and successful approaches to getting young people to engage with the Reading Well for young people books. The school created a wellbeing corner in the library; selected a 'book of the week'; promoted the scheme to the whole school to create inclusivity; put on wellbeing events; created a staff reading challenge; and provided young people the opportunity to review the titles for their peers. One of the key ways the school engaged young people in the programme was the identifications of champions within the school across all levels of the structure, involving heads of year, heads of literacy, library staff and pastoral staff. Students themselves also played roles as champions for the scheme to their peers. Giving both the staff and students the knowledge and understanding of the book list then allowed for them to promote it across the whole of the student and staff body. The report also highlighted the importance of a whole-school approach to introducing the book list, as opposed to targeting it at students who are either diagnosed with or vulnerable to mental health conditions. This approached encouraged widespread discussion about mental health and helped to destigmatize mental health as an 'issue' through the student population.

The report also outlined the key positive impacts of the scheme that were identified during the research:

- improved awareness, knowledge and understanding of mental health conditions
- improved emotional and mental wellbeing, specifically relating to confidence, self-esteem, hope, isolation and emotional intelligence
- changes in behaviour and improved relationships
- normalizing and destigmatizing mental health discussions.

The report outlined that one of the main impacts of the scheme was improved awareness, knowledge and understanding of mental health conditions in the young people. For some participants, reading particular books appeared to help them face their own situation. Sometimes this was because of the information, tips and further sources of help provided by the books; other times, it was the realization that they were not alone with their particular mental health condition. One young person explained simply, 'It just made me feel like if it ever did happen to me or something like that happened there was always something there or someone there to help you.'

The impact on behaviour and discussions around mental health was also a key outcome of the research. From the adult stakeholder perspective, the most reported outcome of the scheme was an increase in interactions and discussions related to mental health. This increase in discussions on mental health that were observed by the adult stakeholders was confirmed by the young people who reported that they had more confidence to talk about what they were feeling as a result of the scheme: 'I think it made me a bit more confident to talk to someone', one young person said. This positive impact was extended to helping young people who do not have a mental health condition have a better understanding of a person who does. Several of the young people reported how having a better understanding of a condition allowed them to change the way they reacted to other people. There were several reports of being more empathetic and understanding towards other people.

The theory of change for the intervention was developed by the researchers at the University of Westminster to show the key resources and mechanisms needed to achieve the above outcomes that had been identified by the interviews and focus groups (Figure 11.1 on the next page).

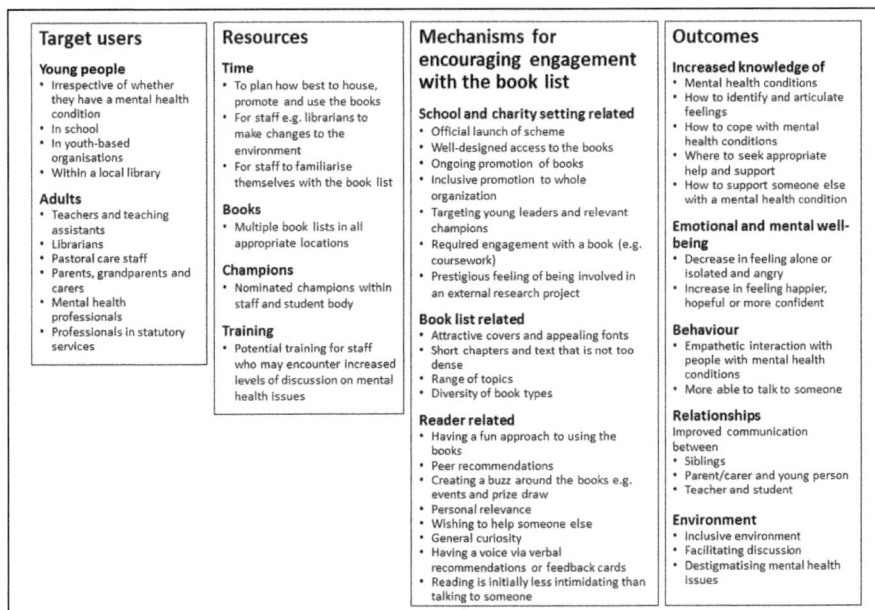

Target users	Resources	Mechanisms for encouraging engagement with the book list	Outcomes
Young people • Irrespective of whether they have a mental health condition • In school • In youth-based organisations • Within a local library **Adults** • Teachers and teaching assistants • Librarians • Pastoral care staff • Parents, grandparents and carers • Mental health professionals • Professionals in statutory services	**Time** • To plan how best to house, promote and use the books • For staff e.g. librarians to make changes to the environment • For staff to familiarise themselves with the book list **Books** • Multiple book lists in all appropriate locations **Champions** • Nominated champions within staff and student body **Training** • Potential training for staff who may encounter increased levels of discussion on mental health issues	**School and charity setting related** • Official launch of scheme • Well-designed access to the books • Ongoing promotion of books • Inclusive promotion to whole organization • Targeting young leaders and relevant champions • Required engagement with a book (e.g. coursework) • Prestigious feeling of being involved in an external research project **Book list related** • Attractive covers and appealing fonts • Short chapters and text that is not too dense • Range of topics • Diversity of book types **Reader related** • Having a fun approach to using the books • Peer recommendations • Creating a buzz around the books e.g. events and prize draw • Personal relevance • Wishing to help someone else • General curiosity • Having a voice via verbal recommendations or feedback cards • Reading is initially less intimidating than talking to someone	**Increased knowledge of** • Mental health conditions • How to identify and articulate feelings • How to cope with mental health conditions • Where to seek appropriate help and support • How to support someone else with a mental health condition **Emotional and mental well-being** • Decrease in feeling alone or isolated and angry • Increase in feeling happier, hopeful or more confident **Behaviour** • Empathetic interaction with people with mental health conditions • More able to talk to someone **Relationships** Improved communication between • Siblings • Parent/carer and young person • Teacher and student **Environment** • Inclusive environment • Facilitating discussion • Destigmatising mental health issues

Figure 11.1 *Theory of change for Shelf Help in a school and charity environment*

The learning going forward

The Reading Agency and SCL hope to continue to embed the Reading Well for young people scheme at the heart of communities and support libraries to continue to build strong local links. Engaging young people in a reading for wellbeing scheme was a challenge that has most definitely been overcome in the ongoing success of the scheme. This is principally a result of engaging young people in the development and delivery of the programme, thus giving them real ownership over it.

References

Latimer Group (2015) *Reading Well Youth Insights 26/11/2015*, https://readingagency.org.uk/resources/Latimer%20Reading%20Well%20Youth%20Insight%20Report.pdf.

Mental Health Foundation (2017) *Mental Health Statistics: children and young people*, www.mentalhealth.org.uk/statistics/mental health-statistics-children-and-young-people.

Statista (2017) *Attitudes Towards Reading Among Young People in the United Kingdom (UK) in 2014 and 2015*, www.statista.com/statistics/299035/young-people-s-attitudes-towards-reading-in-the-uk.

Suffolk Libraries UK (2016) *Reading Well Shelf Help for Young People,*
www.youtube.com/watch?v=COtyp-l2iVo.

The Reading Agency (2015) *Reading Well for Young People Consultation,*
https://readingagency.org.uk/resources/2549.

The Reading Agency (2017) *Reading Facts,*
https://readingagency.org.uk/about/impact/002-reading-facts-1.

The Reading Agency and Society of Chief Librarians (2017) *Reading Well Books on
Prescription: evaluation of year 4 – 2016/17,* https://tra-
resources.s3.amazonaws.com/uploads/entries/document/2480/171009_TRA_
RWBoP_Y4_Evaluation_-_Final.pdf.

University of Westminster (2017) *Evaluation of the Reading Well for Young People
Scheme,* http://westminsterresearch.wmin.ac.uk/19856/1/
Reading%20Well%20for%20young%20people%20evaluation.pdf.

12

Bibliotherapy Read Aloud groups with native and non-native speakers

Kate Gielgud

Introduction

This chapter shares observations made during six years facilitating two Read Aloud bibliotherapy groups in public libraries in the London borough of Westminster. One is an ESOL (English for Speakers of Other Languages) group, while the other has a majority of highly educated native English speakers. Comparing the experiences of these two groups is potentially valuable as, to date, there has been very little research, and relatively few practical examples, of bibliotherapy specifically with migrant communities (Te Pou o Te Whakaaro Nui, 2010).

In March 2010, Westminster Libraries gained funding from the then Westminster Primary Care Trust to deliver an initiative to address health inequalities in the borough and it was decided that Shared Reading would be part of this project. A health information co-ordinator (HIC) was recruited and trained as a shared reading facilitator, alongside an experienced public librarian. Three Shared Reading, or Read Aloud, groups were subsequently started in library settings, including the group at Paddington Library discussed below. In September 2011, I was appointed as the new HIC and took over two of the existing groups, while the librarian continued to facilitate the third group. Within a few months, a fourth group was started by the HIC. Initially, this was advertised as a Read Aloud group for those with English as an additional language. This group meets at Church Street Library. The Church Street area of Westminster has a wide cultural mix, with a large community of non-English speakers and high levels of health inequalities.

This chapter discusses the Paddington and Church Street Read Aloud groups, exploring differences between the two. This includes a discussion of who joins the groups and their motivations for doing so, the types of texts read and the ways in which the groups are facilitated. The chapter starts, however, with an overview of the key features of Shared Reading.

The format of the groups

The Reader launched its 'Get into Reading' initiative in 2008. The Shared Reading approach designed by The Reader is described as, 'a simple idea that changes lives'. By bringing people together to read great literature aloud we are improving wellbeing, reducing social isolation and building stronger communities across the UK and beyond' (www.thereader.org.uk). Typically, a Shared Reading group meets once a week at the same time on the same day and usually in the same place. The meetings last between 90 minutes and two hours, although some groups, such as those for individuals living with dementia, may be shorter. Free tea, coffee and small snacks are provided. The group is led by a Reader-trained facilitator, or Reader Leader, who provides material to be read aloud and facilitates discussion around this material.

The material is generally agreed to be 'great', or at least 'good' literature. It can be in the form of a short story, but once they have been together for a time, many groups choose a novel together that is read aloud in instalments within the group setting. 'Great literature' is generally agreed to be written material which achieves a lasting place in our culture. It is literature that can inspire, teach the power of language and help us to connect to our fellow human beings. Examples of 'great or good literature' might include *The Great Gatsby* by F. Scott Fitzgerald, *Oliver Twist* by Charles Dickens, *Pride and Prejudice* by Jane Austen and *Good Morning Midnight* by Jean Rhys.

In Read Aloud groups, participants explore the journey and experiences of the characters depicted in the book by reading aloud and then discussing what has been read. The facilitator starts the reading aloud and then pauses to invite any comments or observations on what has been read. Group members then continue this process with the facilitator guiding. The final 20–30 minutes of a session is usually spent reading a poem aloud. The poem can be linked to the material read earlier or to current events. Group members do not have to prepare anything in advance, an important advantage for those who may struggle to read a text in English.

The groups operate in a boundaried way, with general principles of respect, such as: arriving on time; listening to each other; having one conversation at a time; and respecting different views and beliefs. The facilitator guides the group bringing attention back to the text so that the focus does not settle on one person and no one gets to 'hold court'. That being said, open sharing and a certain amount of disclosure is sometimes appropriate; the level of this disclosure is usually set out through a group agreement.

The Read Aloud groups are considered to have an 'underlying therapeutic value'. This means that the benefits to the regular group members can be gleaned from what they say about their experiences in the groups and what they take from the group in terms of confidence, support and knowledge. In a library setting, however, there is no formal therapeutic contract and no formal records kept with regard to an individual's wellbeing. Nevertheless, the facilitator takes note of what happens to the group members if they share it with them. In addition, the group setting provides an opportunity to explore other potentially beneficial health, library and community initiatives.

Group members and their motivations for attending

The fact that groups take place within a public library and are open to all means that members can join with very different motivations and expectations of the group. When the new HIC joined the service in late October 2011, the Paddington Library group already had a loyal following of between eight and twelve regular attendees, and the number remained fairly consistent over the next five years. The majority of the group were female and aged over 55. Most were middle-class and highly educated; they had retired from careers in teaching, science, administration and publishing. Although the majority of the group were native English speakers and highly literate, it was advertised as an open group, so from time to time, a non-native English speaker would join, although they would typically only stay for a short period. For example, other members have included a French woman and a Brazilian-Portuguese man, both of whom were keen to improve their English.

Most of the core members of the group said that the main reason they came to the group was because they loved books and reading. Several are confident at reading aloud and also enjoy explaining vocabulary and meaning to any non-native speakers in the group. They also enjoy sharing their knowledge about the lives of the authors and comparing styles of writing. However, they initially showed a certain reticence when it came to group discussions, preferring to stick closely to the more literary aspects of what was read, rather than going deeper into the emotions of a text. For the first two years, there was little, if any, personal disclosure and, as a facilitator, I noted that a polite veil was frequently drawn before any deeper discussions could arise. In late

2013, however, a new member joined after a libraries outreach visit to the local rough sleepers' hostel. Harold started coming to the library every day and sitting reading near where the Shared Reading group meet. We invited him to join the group and take advantage of the free tea and biscuits. After that, he attended every week, often helping to set up the tables and put out the chairs. He did not want to read aloud, but he did make comments from time to time and shared the fact that he had been in prison and had an issue with alcohol. Harold joining the group seemed to mark a turning point; it was impossible to simply ignore his disclosures about his past and current circumstances. The group had to adjust to a greater degree of personal disclosure and started to express concern and think about ways in which they might help Harold.

The Church Street group is very different from the Paddington group in terms of its membership and participants' motivations for joining. It started at the end of 2011 with just three regular members, including two Arabic-speaking women keen to improve their English. Their main motivation for joining the group was to become more proficient in spoken English in order to improve their circumstances. One of the women, Asya, was attending the reading group with the permission of her husband, Faisel; she explained he expected her to use her improved English skills in order to get a job. After a few months, Faisel started coming to the group as well to 'check it out'. Asya had spoken of him as being proficient in English; while this turned out not to be the case, he was a very confident and outgoing personality. Eventually, Asya stopped coming to the group as her expectations in terms of becoming more fluent in English were not met; it became apparent that she wanted to spend time unpicking the grammar in texts, rather than the ideas contained in the stories. However, Faisel was intrigued; he enjoyed the social aspect of the group and continued to attend the group for three and half years.

Gradually, group membership built up to between seven and ten attendees per week, the majority being men and speakers of English as an additional language. There is no doubt that free fresh coffee was a great incentive and the fact that one male Arabic speaker was already coming encouraged others. The men from Iraq, Egypt and Sudan said they were attracted to the prospect of civilized discussion as a way of improving their English. One of the Arabic speakers, Abdul, originally from Egypt, invited his wife Fathiha and daughter Ramina to join and they have both become regular attendees too. Both experience health issues: Fathiha has Parkinson's disease and Ramina lives with muscular dystrophy and is a wheelchair user. This group is not limited to speakers of other languages however, and over time, other members have joined who are native English speakers.

Texts used in the groups

The initial material for the both groups was taken from 'A Little Aloud', an anthology of short stories paired with accompanying poems. This collection was devised for The Reader and is popular with newly trained facilitators. Over time, however, as the groups became more established, they started to read longer texts.

In 2013, the Paddington Library group started to read books in weekly instalments rather than a short story every session. Books read included: *The Island of Dr Moreau* by H. G. Wells, *Candide* by Voltaire, *Cider with Rosie* by Laurie Lee, *The Painted Veil* by W. Somerset Maugham, as well as modern authors, such as Gillian Slovo's *Ten Days*, about the 2010 riots in London. We also read *After the Funeral* by Agatha Christie. There was some debate within the group regarding the status of this book 'great literature' or even 'good literature', but it was accepted to be 'a classic'.

Changes to membership of a Read Aloud group can have an impact on the choice of texts read. For example, the Paddington Library group was joined by an elderly couple in their 80s: Marguerite, who has Alzheimer's, and Holden, her husband and carer. Marguerite enjoyed the reading group and was able to follow parts of the stories and comment on them, but sometimes she would stare blankly into space as the group went on around her. Working with a more mixed group, some of whom had cognitive impairment, meant the choice of material had to alter to reflect that. I found that well known texts with simple themes, such as the short stories of Joanne Harris or 'Daffodils' by Wordsworth, worked best.

In the case of the Church Street group, longer texts are read slowly, over the course of a number of months. *Down and Out in Paris and London* by George Orwell was a popular book with the group in 2015 and more recently, the group has spent almost a year reading *Oliver Twist* by Charles Dickens. All the texts used have been written in English, although we used some translated texts. *A Season of Migration to the North* by Tayeb Salih and the short story *Two Words* by Isabel Allende worked particularly well. Reading aloud these types of original texts containing strong social commentary and/or universal human themes seems to help people pause before responding and allow themselves to be genuinely moved. The texts allow participants to give deeper thought and voice to what it might be like for someone 'other' than themselves and, in this way, come to an understanding of their situations, values and beliefs in a way that allows them to share insights honestly with the group.

A key factor in the success of the Church Street group is the facilitators' continued insistence that no simplified versions of texts be used in the group settings. At one point, it was suggested that it would be easier to use simplified 'readers', as the majority of the group are not native English speakers. Readers are used to support people with learning difficulties and for speakers of English as an additional language. They offer a simplified version of the story with any complex English grammar and vocabulary edited out. However, we decided not to use readers as we feel that the original texts provide a far richer experience for group members. It is true that some of the vocabulary, references and ideas never become completely clear for some of the attendees, but the fact they are given the opportunity to tackle a complete text means the capabilities of the group are not judged or subject to assumptions as to perceived ability or potential. The success of this approach is demonstrated by the fact that some participants want to return to the texts at a later date or in their own time. I would argue that immersion in the original texts provides richer cultural and historical references as well as a window onto, and involvement with, complex human interactions, responses and dilemmas.

Changes in group facilitation

During 2017, Westminster Libraries underwent a period of restructure and the funding of the Read Aloud bibliotherapy groups was in question for a time. However, despite this, both the Paddington and Church Street groups have continued to meet without an official facilitator. They have been, effectively, 'running themselves' and are potentially teaching us a lot about how to sustain the model. In particular, their experiences give an indication of which groups are likely to need more skilled 'leading' to continue working and which may be able to operate without a trained facilitator at each session. Long-standing member Mabel is leading the Paddington Library group with the help of a relatively new member, Jonathan. At Church Street, Betsy and Abdul have been taking it in turns to run the group. A significant difference between using trained group leaders and an informal arrangement where a nominated group member acts as the unofficial leader is that the unofficial group leaders do not have to prepare the provided text. A trained Read Aloud leader, whether they are a staff member or a volunteer, will prepare the text before the session. This will help non-native English speakers, as well other more vulnerable groups, such as those living with cognitive impairment, to engage more fully in the group discussion. The impact of the lack of a trained facilitator quickly became apparent at Church Street, where many non-native English speakers stopped attending regularly for a time.

Read Aloud groups are a valuable part of the library offer in these changing times. I believe they need care and maintenance to continue to be effective: this includes investment by, and joint working from, libraries, councils, public health and clinical commissioning groups in terms of training and support of volunteer facilitators. A well-established Read Aloud group primarily motivated to meet to combat isolation, such as that at Paddington Library, may be able to meet on its own, providing there is practical support from the library and input and interest from a trained facilitator at intervals. However, maintaining a group, even for a short period, without a trained facilitator is more challenging for groups with a high proportion of non-native speakers and other more vulnerable participants. Although one of the unofficial leaders at Church Street has begun to prepare texts prior to sessions, the ideal is to have more trained volunteer Reader Leaders with experience in the fields of mental health, arts therapies, and of course literature. Trained volunteers will be better equipped to prepare for sessions effectively and facilitate discussions in a way that allows everyone to feel involved. Our intention, therefore, is for every Westminster Libraries Shared Reading group to have a trained volunteer Reader Leader and I am confident that the Church Street ESOL group will recover in strength once this is back in place.

Conclusion

The Church Street Shared Reading group has now met every week for five and a half years, continuing through different facilitators and a library restructure. Embracing challenge is an important part of the success and survival of a Read Aloud group: challenge in terms of the material and in terms of human connection. Overcoming barriers of language and prejudice through mutual appreciation of literature and the basic simple idea of coming together on a regular basis has made the Church Street Read Aloud group a success story for participants past and present.

In conclusion, Read Aloud groups can bring together people of all ages, abilities and ethnicities, leading them out of isolation and enabling them to access knowledge and heritage along with providing companionship and nurturing self-care skills. However, it is important to be clear about the purpose of a Read Aloud group, so that participants are not left disappointed. Non-native speakers who wish to improve their English through learning about grammar are unlikely to find their needs met through a Read Aloud group. They may be better suited to classes run in partnership with adult education services; Westminster Libraries hosts such classes free to unwaged residents as part of its 'Read Learn Connect' offer that embraces the more practical aspects of education along with a supportive exploration of cultural heritage and collaborative innovation. However, for non-native speakers looking for social connections and more informal opportunities for discussion that may improve their understanding of English literature and language, participation in a Read Aloud group is likely to provide significant benefits.

Reference

Te Pou o te Whakaaro Nui (2010) *Therapies for Refugees, Asylum Seekers and New Migrants: best and promising practice guide for mental health and addiction services,* www.mentalhealth.org.nz/assets/ResourceFinder/Talking-Therapies-for-Refugees-Asylum-Seekers-and-New-Migrants.pdf.

13

Promoting student wellbeing through a student success collection

Elena Azadbakht and Tracy Englert

Introduction

In the summer of 2016, we created a Student Success Collection (SSC) at the University of Southern Mississippi's main library in Hattiesburg, Mississippi, USA. This niche collection is comprised of over 300 titles related to student success, broadly defined, and is displayed in the Cook Library lobby adjacent to the campus Starbucks coffee shop. Items in the SSC encompass a variety of topics, such as study skills, writing manuals and time management, as well as career and vocational development, personal growth and development, health and wellbeing and other issues related to student life. Also included are support materials for instructors, covering topics from excellence in teaching to professional growth. Quality instruction is, after all, a component of student success.

We were inspired to create our Student Success Collection in part by an article by Ke, Greive and Vaughn (2015) discussing a collection of books on developing academic skills that were relocated to the University of Houston library's busy ground floor, thereby increasing their visibility. We were also motivated by our university's recent Student Success Initiative and, in our effort to identify ways in which Cook Library could play a part in this push, we recalled book displays we had previously pulled together on topics related to some aspects of student success. Our general collection included many titles related to student success, but these were spread out all throughout the stacks according to the Library of Congress Classification System. We had given out a printed bibliography of these items at student orientations and other outreach events. When our institution's president started a book club in the summer of 2015, we created a tailored list of leadership and academic success items in support of it. These projects served as the springboard for our permanent SSC.

This article describes the background to this initiative; examines practical aspects such as the location of the collection, stock selection and promotion; and finally outlines some possible future directions

Background

Part of being a successful student is dependent on maintaining a healthy body and mind amidst a variety of different stressors. For the purposes of creating this collection, we chose to define health and wellness in a broad way and have selected material aimed at improving all aspects of students' lives. Our particular student population and locality – a diverse group of largely first-generation college students in a region of the USA with traditionally poor health and economic indicators – inspires such an inclusive interpretation of 'success'.

The University of Southern Mississippi is a public institution founded in 1910 that is classified as having a 'higher research activity' by the Carnegie Foundation (2015). It has a total enrolment of nearly 15,000 students, comprised of new first-time undergraduates as well as transfers from Mississippi community colleges (The University of Southern Mississippi Office of Institutional Research, 2017). Many of these students face significant challenges. According to the National Center for Education Statistics (2015), approximately 78% of our undergraduates received some form of need-based financial aid during the 2015–16 academic year. As of autumn 2016, about 82% of our undergraduate students were residents of Mississippi. Roughly a third of these students are from historically underserved ethnic/racial minority groups and nearly two-thirds are women. Only about half of University of Southern Mississippi undergraduates are expected to graduate within in six years, based on information from the University's Office of Institutional Research (The University of Southern Mississippi Office of Institutional Research, 2016).

Mississippi is a rural state in the south-central USA and has traditionally faced many challenges. It not only has a high rate of poverty (as compared to other states), but is consistently ranked as the lowest in the nation on a variety of health and wellness measures. The 2016 American Community Survey estimates that 20.8% of the state's population currently lives in poverty (United States Census Bureau, 2016). According to the Centers for Disease Control and Prevention, in 2015 Mississippi led the nation in deaths caused by heart disease, stroke, and diabetes. The state also had the second-highest teen birth rate (mothers aged 15–19) and the highest preterm birth rate in that year (Centers for Disease Control/National Center for Health Statistics, 2017). The University of Southern Mississippi is located in Forrest County, which has an adult obesity rate of roughly 34% and increasing rates of sexually transmitted infections (County Health Rankings & Roadmaps, 2017).

In a review of the literature on student success in academic libraries, much of the focus has been on information literacy instruction and how students' use of library services and collections correlates to their academic performance. Likewise, while there are many studies that consider the development, use and the effectiveness of bibliotherapy as an intervention, none explicitly address the role of bibliotherapy in relation to student success. Two articles, however, feature collections similar to the one we have created at the University of Southern Mississippi.

In 'Improving Retention: leveraging collections for student success,' Ke and colleagues discuss how the University of Houston library relocated key titles on academic success to a high-traffic area on the building's ground floor. They observe that the '[s]tudents who need these types of books the most can often feel the least comfortable navigating the stacks' (Ke, Greive and Vaughn, 2015, 26). The authors also mention that items relating to mental health and wellness were being considered for their collection.

More than 25 years before, Allen and Workman (1989) had described the creation of a 'self-management lab' comprised of a variety of self-help materials (pamphlets, books, audiovisual resources, etc.) that students could browse through on the main floor of the undergraduate library at the University of Illinois at Urbana-Champaign. While the idea for the collection itself originated with the institution's counselling centre and Health Service Health Education department, they brought the library in as a partner because of its 'broadly defined education mission as well as a reputation for innovation' (Allen and Workman, 1989, 106). The undergraduate library provided an ideal space for the self-management lab and was also able to help purchase the materials for it. The lab was staffed by counselling centre personnel during key hours, and the authors estimate that these staff members assisted more than 2400 students during the 1987–88 academic year (Allen and Workman, 1989, 107).

Locating the SSC

Once we began to consider the possibility of establishing a small collection focused on student success, the Research Services and Access Services units within Cook Library worked together to decide on a location for the collection and to determine circulation loan periods for the materials. The SSC was ultimately placed on shelving in the lobby of Cook Library directly outside of the Starbucks coffee shop located there, which is a very high-traffic area. Many students, faculty and staff members from across campus begin their days by coming by the Starbucks for coffee, tea and treats, and they often meet with one another in or near this area of our library.

We opted to repurpose shelving left over from our popular reading display, which was also housed in this corner of the Cook Library lobby. We created new signage with the help of the University Libraries' Assistant to the Dean for Publicity and Outreach to delineate the two collections. While the majority of the items in the general collection circulate for 30 days (with even longer loan periods for faculty and graduate students), the books in the SSC were all given a loan period of 14 days to increase access to more students, faculty and staff. The books are organized using the Library of Congress Classification System, like the majority of Cook Library materials, with several of the most popular and aesthetically pleasing titles displayed on book stands at roughly eye-level on top of the shelving.

Selecting stock

Initially, the SSC consisted entirely of titles drawn from Cook Library's general collection. While we were able to identify around 150 or so quality books that we thought would benefit our students and faculty, we also found many books that were either out of date or not reflective of the needs of current students. Since our project was in support of the university's Student Success Initiative, we applied for, and were awarded, a small grant from the Friends of the University Libraries organization to purchase new titles to enhance and enrich the collection. We decided to primarily choose titles from the following categories:

- academic writing
- study skills
- academic integrity (especially plagiarism)
- time management
- stress management
- diet and nutrition (including cookbooks)
- exercise
- mental health (e.g., managing anxiety and depression)
- sexual health

- interpersonal issues (e.g., relationships with roommates)
- gay, lesbian, bisexual, transgender, and questioning (LGBTQ) issues
- financial literacy
- career resources
- motivational nonfiction (primarily memoirs).

In order to develop a relevant and current collection that appeals to, and meets the needs of, students and faculty, we carefully selected titles from reviews, suggested titles lists and topical subject coverage guides, such as the American Psychological Association's 'Life Tools: books for the general public' series; the American Library Association GLBT Round Table's 'Over the Rainbow Books';[1] and *The Chronicle of Higher Education's* 'Selected Books on Higher Education'. We also ordered titles featured in popular TED Talks as well as those written by guest lecturers and other visitors to campus. We researched best-sellers and read blog posts and short informal articles on sites such as ProfHacker[2] and GradHacker.[3]

We consulted several resources in our effort to procure books on diet, nutrition, exercise, and fitness that would appeal to college students. Although we wanted to provide our campus community with trustworthy sources of information, we also sought more 'popular' titles for the SSC rather than the material students and faculty would encounter in their coursework and research. This approach led us to titles such as *The Healthy College Cookbook* (Nimetz, Stanley and Starr, 2009); *The Smart Student's Guide to Healthy Living: how to survive stress, late nights, and the college cafeteria* (Smith, Fada and Smith, 2006); and *The 'Go Ask Alice' Book of Answers: a guide to good physical, sexual, and emotional health* (Columbia University, 2008).

We worked with our colleagues in Access Services and Technical Services to facilitate the creation of the SSC. The titles we had identified had to be pulled, labelled and re-shelved. In the University Libraries' online catalogue, a location called Cook Library Display was created. For physical processing of the items, a bright yellow label was created that said 'student success' and this was affixed to the spine of the items (see Figure 13.1 on the next page). Due to the constraints of the integrated library system (ILS) we use, it was deemed infeasible to create a separate location scope. Thus, in order to create a list, we established a workaround and listed all the SSC items as 'on (course) reserve' in a fake course called 'student success.' Items we purchased using the Friends of the University Libraries grant we received were given a note in the catalogue record, 'purchased by a grant from Friends of University Libraries'.

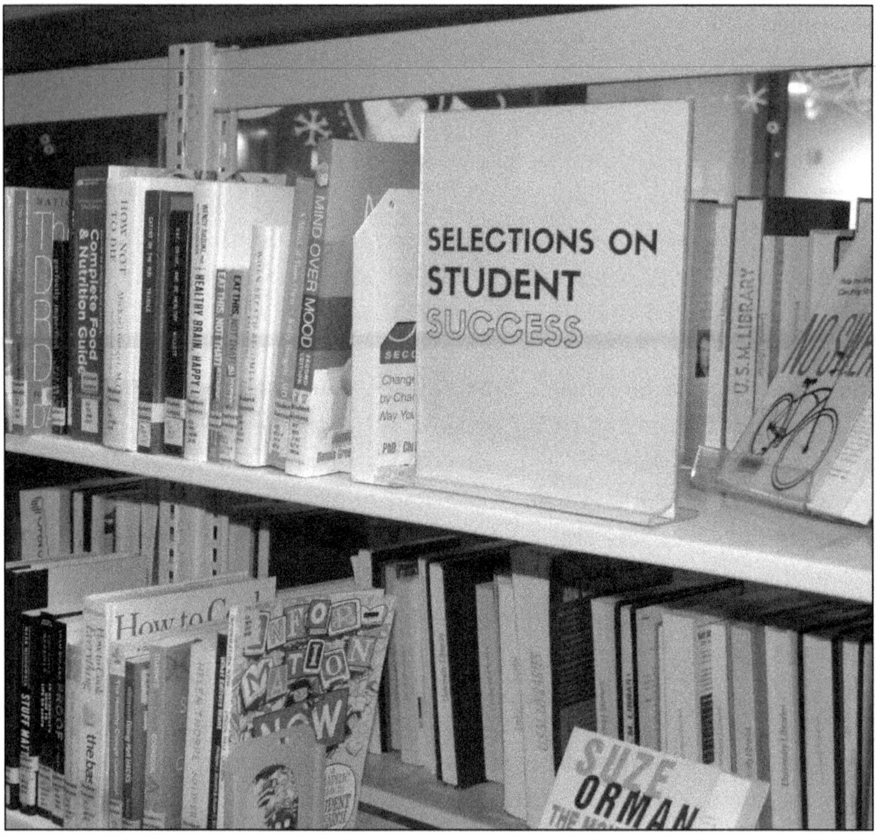

Figure 13.1 *The Student Success Collection*

Promoting the SSC

In terms of promoting the SSC, we utilized several different venues. We already maintain dozens of online LibGuides on a variety of topics, so it made sense to use the popular SpringShare product for this project as well. We created two LibGuides for our two distinct audiences of students and their instructors. The former we called 'Student Success' and the latter became 'Faculty Development.' This not only provided us with a way to promote the items in the SSC online, but also enabled the inclusion of relevant e-books and other electronic resources that have no physical counterpart (such as a link out to our *The Chronicle of Higher Education* subscription on the 'Faculty Development' guide).

We worked again with the University Libraries' Assistant to the Dean for Publicity and Outreach and the graphic designers at our institution's Office of University Communications to create colourful two-sided rack cards that describe the collection and advertise the two corresponding LibGuides. These were passed out at New Faculty Orientation and other campus outreach events. We have also reached out to our new Faculty Development Center and the Southern Miss Student Success Initiative to help us alert the campus community to the SSC.

The SSC's location has served as a key promotional tool. Many new student orientation sessions and library instruction sessions for classes, such as the required introductory composition course, begin in the Cook Library lobby, so it has been easy to draw the visiting students' attention to the collection at those times. Moreover, most campus tour groups consisting of prospective students and their parents include a stop in the library lobby, where the SSC is now a prominent feature.

SSC usage

It has been challenging to gauge the SSC's appeal. A recent circulation usage report revealed that 162 of the items in the SSC have been checked out – roughly half of the collection. Of those, 103 have been checked out more than once. Anecdotally, we have seen many students and faculty browse the collection on their way in and out of the Starbucks or while they are waiting for a friend or colleague in the lobby. When we have had reference desk interactions with students in recent months, several have asked for material relating to topics covered by the SSC and it has been easy to simply walk them over to the lobby. Every so often, students will inquire about books they had previously seen displayed but that are currently checked out. Among the five most checked out titles are two explicitly related to health and wellbeing:

- *Sex for Life: from virginity to Viagra, how sexuality changes throughout our lives* (2012) edited by Laura Carpenter and John DeLamater
- *Psychology of Champions: how to win at sports and life with the focus edge of super-athletes* (2008) by James J. Barrell and David Ryback.

Interestingly, since the time of its inception, several titles have been checked out and not returned, which we feel is some measure of success. We have acquired replacement titles, but it has sometimes taken some time to ensure that titles slated for the SSC do in fact end up there and not elsewhere in the stacks.

Future directions

Although budgetary constraints have made it more difficult to find the funds for expanding niche collections, we hope that we will gradually pull more items into the SSC. The University of Southern Mississippi plans to place even more of a focus on student success endeavours in the near future and we believe that the SSC should play a role in supporting these projects. As such, local funding opportunities may serve as a means of further developing the collection. We are also digging deeper into the existing general collection for titles that relate to student success or faculty development in some way – titles that we may have overlooked in our initial search. Likewise, academic departments may request books that have broad appeal and could be added to the SSC.

The SSC is also a possible vehicle for intra-university collaboration and targeted outreach. For instance, the Office of New Student and Retention Programs on our campus has organized a 'Student Success Series' of workshops and events in recent semesters that focus on various aspects of being a successful college student. We are thinking of tailoring our LibGuide to mirror some of the topics covered in the series and promoting the SSC and LibGuide at these events. Another example is 'Stress Less Week,' which is an annual event organized by the university's Office of Health Promotion that aims to help students deal with the stress of exams in healthy ways. Cook Library already has a 'Stress Relief Area' of colouring sheets and puzzles that we set up in a corner during Stress Less Week, but we are considering ways in which we might highlight the stress management books in the SSC during this time as well.

Another possible use for the SSC is as the starting point for a 'pop-up library,' an event in which library staff set up a temporary space elsewhere on a campus, effectively bringing the library to where the students are (Barnett, Bull and Cooper, 2016; Davis et al., 2015). Often, pop-up libraries consist of a few staff with some technology and several books that can be checked out to patrons then and there. Hosting a pop-up library during a campus event would give us a way to showcase certain titles in the SSC as well as promote library services more generally. We think events being planned by campus groups such as the Southern Miss PRISM LGBTQ Office, the campus fitness centre/gymnasium, the student health centre and campus career services are venues that tie in with some aspect of the SSC.

Conclusion

Overall, we have been pleased with the response from our campus community, especially other academic support units. We anticipate that many promising opportunities for collaboration will arise as a result of the SSC. The usage statistics were more impressive than we imagined they would be. While usage of our print collection has been decreasing, as is the case at many libraries, use of the SSC has been fairly robust for a collection of its size and scope. The challenge going forward will be to find ways of maintaining the collection, and even expanding it, while still keeping it usable and relevant to our students, faculty and staff.

Notes

1 www.glbtrt.ala.org/overtherainbow.
2 www.chronicle.com/blogs/profhacker.
3 www.insidehighered.com/blogs/gradhacker.

References

Allen, D. R. and Workman, G. (1989) An Interdepartmental Self-management Lab: a self-help approach to student development, *Journal of Counseling & Development*, **68** (1), 106–8.

Barnett, J., Bull, S. and Cooper, H. (2016) Pop-up Library at the University of Birmingham: extending the reach of an academic library by taking 'the library' to the students, *New Review of Academic Librarianship*, **22** (2/3), 112–31.

Carnegie Foundation (2015) *Classification of Institutions of Higher Education*, http://carnegieclassifications.iu.edu/listings.php.

Centers for Disease Control and Prevention/National Center for Health Statistics (2017) *Stats of the State of Mississippi*, www.cdc.gov/nchs/pressroom/states/mississippi/mississippi.htm.

Columbia University (2008) *The 'Go Ask Alice' Book of Answers: a guide to good physical, sexual, and emotional health*, Paw Prints.

County Health Rankings & Roadmaps (2017) *Forrest County, Mississippi*, www.countyhealthrankings.org/app/mississippi/2017/rankings/forrest/county/outcomes/overall/snapshot.

Davis, A., Rice, C., Spagnolo, D., Struck, J. and Bull, S. (2015) Exploring Pop-up Libraries in Practice, *Australian Library Journal*, **64** (2), 94–104.

Ke, I., Greive, K. and Vaughn, P. (2015) Improving Retention: leveraging collections for student success, *American Libraries*, **46** (9/10), 26.

National Center for Education Statistics (2015) *College Navigator*, https://nces.ed.gov/collegenavigator.

Nimetz, A., Stanley, J. and Starr, E. (2009) *The Healthy College Cookbook*, 2nd edn, Storey Publishing LLC.

Smith, M. J., Fada, R. D. and Smith, F. (2006) *The Smart Student's Guide to Healthy Living: how to survive stress, late nights, and the college cafeteria*, New Harbinger Publications.

United States Census Bureau (2016) *U.S. Census Bureau QuickFacts Selected: Mississippi*, www.census.gov/quickfacts/MS.

The University of Southern Mississippi Office of Institutional Research (2016) *Quick Facts – Fall 2016*, www.usm.edu/sites/default/files/groups/office-institutional-research/pdf/quick_facts_fall_2016.pdf.

The University of Southern Mississippi Office of Institutional Research (2017) *Fall 2017 Snapshot*, www.usm.edu/institutional-research.

Index